Study Guide for

Fundamental Nursing Skills and Concepts

TENTH EDITION

BARBARA K. TIMBY, RN, BC, BSN, MA
Nursing Professor
Glen Oaks Community College
Centreville, Michigan

 Wolters Kluwer | Lippincott Williams & Wilkins
Health
Philadelphia · Baltimore · New York · London
Buenos Aires · Hong Kong · Sydney · Tokyo

Product Manager: Annette Ferran
Design Coordinator: Joan Wendt
Illustration Coordinator: Brett MacNaughton
Manufacturing Coordinator: Karin Duffield
Prepress Vendor: Aptara, Inc.

9 8 7 6 5 4 3 2 1

Printed in the United States of America

ISBN: 978-1-4511-5167-1

Care has been taken to confirm the accuracy of the information presented and to describe generally accepted practices. However, the authors, editors, and publisher are not responsible for errors or omissions or for any consequences from application of the information in this book and make no warranty, expressed or implied, with respect to the currency, completeness, or accuracy of the contents of the publication. Application of this information in a particular situation remains the professional responsibility of the practitioner; the clinical treatments described and recommended may not be considered absolute and universal recommendations.

The authors, editors, and publisher have exerted every effort to ensure that drug selection and dosage set forth in this text are in accordance with the current recommendations and practice at the time of publication. However, in view of ongoing research, changes in government regulations, and the constant flow of information relating to drug therapy and drug reactions, the reader is urged to check the package insert for each drug for any change in indications and dosage and for added warnings and precautions. This is particularly important when the recommended agent is a new or infrequently employed drug.

Some drugs and medical devices presented in this publication have Food and Drug Administration (FDA) clearance for limited use in restricted research settings. It is the responsibility of the health care provider to ascertain the FDA status of each drug or device planned for use in his or her clinical practice.

LWW.COM

Preface

This study guide was developed to accompany the tenth edition of *Fundamental Nursing Skills and Concepts* by Barbara K. Timby. The study guide is designed to help you practice and retain the knowledge you've gained from the textbook, and it is structured to integrate that knowledge and give you a basis for applying it in your nursing practice. The following types of exercises are provided in each chapter of the study guide.

ASSESSING YOUR UNDERSTANDING

The first section of each study guide chapter concentrates on the basic information of the textbook chapter and helps you to remember key concepts, vocabulary, and principles.

- Fill in the Blanks
  Fill-in-the-blank exercises help you to recall important chapter information. They also test key chapter information, encouraging you to recall key points.
- Labeling
  Labeling exercises are used where you need to remember certain visual representations of the concepts presented in the textbook.
- Match the Following
  Matching questions test your knowledge of the definition of key terms.
- Sequencing
  Sequencing exercises ask you to remember particular sequences or orders, for instance testing processes and prioritizing nursing actions.

- Short Answers
  Short answer questions cover facts, concepts, procedures, and principles of the chapter. These questions ask you to recall information as well as demonstrate your comprehension of the information.
- Crossword Puzzles
  Crossword Puzzles also cover important facts, concepts, procedures, and principles of the chapter in a diverting exercise.

APPLYING YOUR KNOWLEDGE

The second section of each Study Guide chapter consists of case study based exercises that ask you to begin to apply the knowledge you've gained from the textbook chapter and reinforced in the first section of the Study Guide chapter. A case study scenario based on the chapter's content is presented, and then you are asked to answer some questions, in writing, related to the case study. The questions cover the following areas:

- Assessment
- Planning Nursing Care
- Communication
- Reflection

PRACTICING FOR NCLEX

The third and final section of the study chapters helps you practice NCLEX-style questions while further reinforcing the knowledge you have been gaining and testing for yourself through the textbook chapter and the first two sections of the study guide chapter. In keeping with the NCLEX, the questions presented are multiple-choice and scenario based, asking you to reflect, consider, and apply what you know and to choose the best answer out of those offered.

ANSWER KEY

The answers for all of the exercises and questions in the study guide are provided online at thePoint, so you can assess your own learning as you complete each chapter.

We hope you will find this study guide to be helpful and enjoyable, and we wish you every success in your studies toward becoming a nurse.

The Publishers

Contents

CHAPTER 1

Nursing Foundations

SECTION I: LEARNING OBJECTIVES

- Name one historical event that led to the demise of nursing in England before the time of Florence Nightingale.
- Identify four reforms for which Florence Nightingale is responsible.
- Describe at least five ways in which early U.S. training schools deviated from those established under the direction of Florence Nightingale.
- Name three ways that nurses used their skills in the early history of U.S. nursing.
- Explain how art, science, and nursing theory have been incorporated into contemporary nursing practice.
- Discuss the evolution of definitions of nursing.
- List four types of educational programs that prepare students for beginning levels of nursing practice.
- Identify at least five factors that influence choice of educational nursing programs.
- State three reasons that support the need for continuing education in nursing.
- List examples of current trends affecting nursing and health care.
- Discuss the shortage of nurses and methods to reduce the crisis.
- Describe four skills that all nurses use in clinical practice.

SECTION II: ASSESSING YOUR UNDERSTANDING

Activity A *Fill in the blanks.*

1. The word _____ is derived from the Latin word *scio*, which means "I know."

2. _____ refers to feeling as emotionally distraught as the client.

3. Nightingale started the first training school for nurses at St. Thomas Hospital in _____.

4. _____ is the ability to perform an act skillfully.

5. American nurses worked alongside physicians in Mobile Army Surgical Hospitals during the _____ War.

6. The word _____ comes from a Greek word that means "vision" and refers to an opinion, belief, or view that explains a process.

7. _____ graduates are a vital link between the registered nurse and unlicensed assistive personnel (UAP).

8. _____ skills are nursing acts that involve collecting data.

9. _____ prepared nurses have the greatest flexibility in qualifying for nursing positions, both staff and managerial.

10. _____ refers to the intuitive awareness of what feeling the client is experiencing.

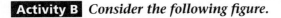

Activity B *Consider the following figure.*

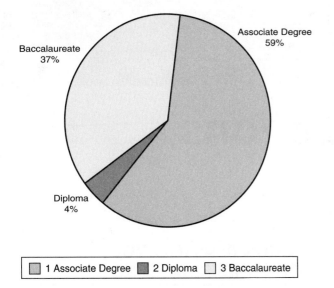

- ☐ 1 Associate Degree ☐ 2 Diploma ☐ 3 Baccalaureate

1. What are the educational options available in a nursing career?

_____

_____

_____

2. What are the factors that affect the choice of a nursing program?

_____

_____

_____

Activity C *Match the types of nursing skills in column A with their description in column B.*

Column A

____ 1. Assessment skills

____ 2. Comforting skills

____ 3. Counseling skills

____ 4. Caring skills

Column B

A. Nursing interventions that restore or maintain a person's health

B. Acts that involve collecting data

C. Interventions that provide stability and security during a health-related crisis

D. Interventions that include communicating with clients and providing emotional support

Activity D *Write the correct sequence of the line of authority and delegation of work in a nursing unit in the boxes provided.*

1. Registered nurse

2. Unlicensed assistive personnel

3. Licensed practical nurse (LPN)

4. Physician

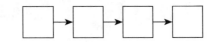

The following are the events related to Florence Nightingale. Arrange the events in chronological order in the boxes provided.

1. Florence Nightingale establishes a training school for nurses in England.

2. Florence Nightingale works with the Institution for the Care of Sick Gentlewomen in Distressed Circumstances.

3. Florence Nightingale works with nursing deaconesses, a Protestant order of women.

4. Florence Nightingale provides nursing care to soldiers during the Crimean War.

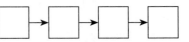

Activity E *Briefly answer the following.*

1. What selection criteria were established by Dorothea Lynde Dix for recruitment of nurses?

_____

_____

_____

2. What is the definition of nursing according to Virginia Henderson?

_____

_____

_____

3. What are the six essential features that characterize nursing?

_____

_____

_____

4. What are the factors that influence the choice of a nursing program?

_____

_____

_____

5. What are the guidelines to be kept in mind while delegating nursing tasks to staff members?

_____

_____

_____

Activity F *Use the clues to complete the crossword puzzle.*

Across

1. Opinion, belief, or view that explains a process; comes from a Greek word that means vision
2. This English word comes from the Latin word *scio*
3. The type of nursing skills or interventions that restore or maintain a person's health
4. Intuitive awareness of what the client is experiencing

Down

5. Famous war that brought nursing into the limelight
6. The type of listening that demonstrates full attention to what is being said, hearing both the content being communicated and the unspoken message

SECTION III: APPLYING YOUR KNOWLEDGE

Activity G *Nursing skills are activities that are unique to the practice of nursing. One of these skills is the counseling skill that the nurse implements during exchanges of information, offering pertinent health teaching and providing emotional support to the clients. Answer the following questions, which involve implementation of nursing skills.*

An 8-year-old boy with a tapeworm infection visits his primary care doctor along with his mother. The mother is worried that her child seems to be weak and is not gaining weight.

1. What nursing skills should the nurse use to provide effective nursing care to this client?

   _____

   _____

   _____

2. What are the advantages of active listening in communicating with a client?

   _____

   _____

   _____

SECTION IV: PRACTICING FOR NCLEX

Activity H *Answer the following questions.*

1. What was the most important nursing contribution of Florence Nightingale and her team of nurses during the Crimean War?

   a. The death rate of soldiers decreased from 60% to 1%

   b. Sanitary conditions for the sick and injured were improved

   c. The soldiers were given hygienic food to eat

   d. Infection and gangrene in the soldiers was controlled

2. A client reports to the primary health care center for his regular checkup. Which of the following activities of the nurse demonstrates the use of assessment skills?

   a. Telling the client to exercise daily

   b. Palpating the abdomen for liver enlargement

   c. Educating the client about the hepatitis B vaccination program

   d. Ensuring that the client is taking his medication regularly

3. A mother is informed by the oncologist that her son has been diagnosed with terminal cancer. What nursing skills should the nurse use to help the mother cope with this news?

   a. Assessment skills

   b. Caring skills

   c. Comforting skills

   d. Counseling skills

4. As a result of diabetic complications, a client has had a leg amputated. The nurse uses empathy to perceive the client's emotional state and need for support. How would empathy help the nurse?

   a. It helps her avoid hurting the client's emotions and feelings unknowingly

   b. It helps her provide effective care while remaining compassionately detached

   c. It helps her provide emotional support to the emotionally unstable client

   d. It helps her counsel the client effectively by suggesting available rehabilitation options

5. A 50-year-old client is admitted to nursing care in an unconscious state. What nursing skills does the nurse demonstrate by interviewing the client's wife?

   a. Counseling skill

   b. Comforting skill

   c. Caring skill

   d. Assessment skill

6. The nurse, after assessing the client's needs, delegates nursing tasks to the nursing staff. Which of the following factors should the nurse keep in mind while delegating the work?

   a. Knowing the unique competencies of the caregiver

   b. Ensuring that care is given to the right client

   c. Confirming that the caregiver is sincere in his or her work

   d. Ensuring that the client deserves the care

7. A nurse delegates the task of changing the colostomy bag of a client to the LPN. The LPN informs the nurse that she has never done the procedure on a client. What should the appropriate action of the nurse be?

   a. Perform the procedure with the LPN and teach her

   b. Request that the LPN refer to the procedure manual

   c. Request that the LPN take the manual along and do the procedure

   d. Request that the LPN observe another LPN who knows the procedure

8. A nurse assigns an LPN to change the position of a comatose client. Which of the following statements demonstrates the correct direction guideline while delegating the nursing task?

   a. "Change the position of the comatose client and report back to me."

   b. "Change the position of the client in cubicle number 3 and give him a back rub."

   c. "Change the position of the client, give him a back rub, and report back to me."

   d. "Change the position of the comatose client in cubicle 3 and give him a back rub."

9. The nurse is caring for a client who is experiencing pain at the surgical incision site during the postoperative period. Which of the following nursing statements would indicate assessment?

   a. "Please take this analgesic medication; it will reduce the pain."

   b. "Can you rate the pain on the pain scale, from 1 to 10?"

   c. "Don't worry; it is the result of surgery; it will subside after some time."

   d. "Guard the incision site with your palm during movements."

10. A client is scheduled to undergo arthroplasty of the knee. On the day of surgery, the client expresses his anxiety, because he is undergoing surgery for the first time. What statement should the nurse use to comfort the client and alleviate his anxiety?

    a. "The operating team is very competent and the surgery has had good outcomes."

    b. "You should not worry; there is always a first time for everything."

    c. "Don't worry; even I underwent the same surgery a few months back."

    d. "There are many people who undergo this surgery without any problem."

11. Several types of programs prepare graduates in registered nursing. Each educational track provides the knowledge and skills for a particular entry level of practice. Which of the following factors affects a student's choice of a nursing program? Select all that apply.

    a. Career goals

    b. Type of training

    c. Length of program

    d. Job availability

    e. Cost involved

12. Nurses use active listening, which facilitates therapeutic interactions. By active listening, the nurses demonstrate full attention to what is being said, hearing both the content being communicated and the unspoken message. Which of the following is an example of active listening? Select all that apply.

    a. The nurse nods her head when the client speaks

    b. The nurse repeats what the client has said

    c. The nurse expresses her own emotions

    d. The nurse observes the client's body language

    e. The nurse relates what he or she is hearing to an incident that happened with her

13. A client reports to the emergency department with pain in the leg as a result of a fall in the garden. The nurse tells the client to describe the incident. Which of the following nursing skills is the nurse using?

   a. Assessment skills

   b. Comforting skills

   c. Counseling skills

   d. Caring skills

14. Shortage of nurses is a major issue today. Which of the following are factors that have contributed to the nursing shortage? Select all that apply.

   a. Increased aging population requiring health care

   b. Limited scope for educational growth

   c. Publicity about mandatory overtime

   d. Heavier workloads and sicker clients

   e. Rigorous training and difficult life

15. A student wishes to pursue a career in nursing. Which of the following nursing programs offers the shortest course in registered nursing?

   a. Graduate nursing programs

   b. Baccalaureate programs

   c. Associate degree programs

   d. Hospital-based diploma programs

CHAPTER 2

Nursing Process

SECTION I: LEARNING OBJECTIVES

- Define the nursing process.
- Describe six characteristics of the nursing process.
- List five steps in the nursing process.
- Identify four sources for assessment data.
- Differentiate between a data base assessment and a focus assessment.
- Distinguish between a nursing diagnosis and a collaborative problem.
- List three parts of a nursing diagnostic statement.
- Describe the rationale for setting priorities.
- Discuss appropriate circumstances for short-term and long-term goals.
- Identify four ways to document a plan of care.
- Describe the information that is documented in reference to the plan of care.
- Discuss three outcomes that result from evaluation.
- Describe the process of concept mapping as an alternative learning strategy for student clinical experiences.

SECTION II: ASSESSING YOUR UNDERSTANDING

Activity A *Fill in the blanks.*

1. A _____ is a set of actions that leads to a particular goal.

2. _____ is the first step in the nursing process.

3. _____ data are observable and measurable facts that are referred to as signs of a disorder.

4. _____ is the primary source for information.

5. _____ is a step in the nursing process that means carrying out the plan of care.

6. A(n) _____ assessment is information that provides more details about specific problems and expands the original data base.

7. _____ refers to the identification of health-related problems.

8. A body temperature measurement is considered _____ data.

9. Problems interfering with the _____ needs of a client have priority over those affecting other levels of needs.

10. _____ problems are physiologic complications that require both nurse- and physician-prescribed interventions.

Activity B *Consider the following figures.*

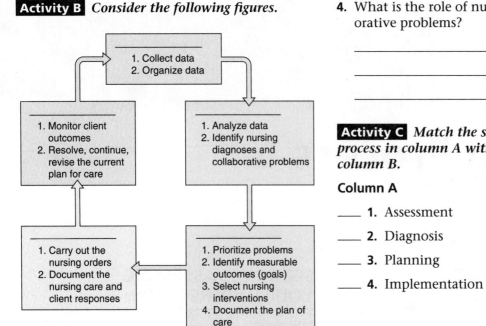

1. List the steps of the nursing process.

_____

_____

_____

2. What are the types of data collected during assessment?

_____

_____

_____

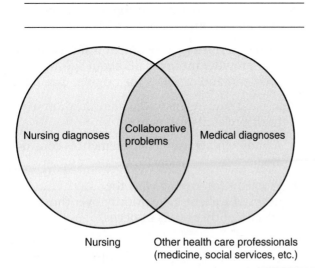

3. What are collaborative problems?

_____

_____

_____

4. What is the role of nurses in managing collaborative problems?

_____

_____

_____

Activity C *Match the steps of the nursing process in column A with its description in column B.*

Column A

____ **1.** Assessment

____ **2.** Diagnosis

____ **3.** Planning

____ **4.** Implementation

Column B

A. Process of carrying out the plan of care

B. Process of prioritizing nursing diagnoses and collaborative problems

C. Systematic collection of facts or data

D. Identification of health-related problems

Activity D *Presented here, in random order, are the steps of the nursing process. Write the correct sequence in the boxes provided below.*

1. Implementation

2. Planning

3. Evaluation

4. Assessment

5. Diagnosis

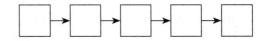

Activity E *Briefly answer the following.*

1. What is meant by the nursing process?

_____

_____

_____

2. What are the characteristics of the nursing process?

_____

_____

_____

3. What are the two types of assessments?

_____

_____

_____

4. What is concept mapping?

_____

_____

_____

5. What are the characteristics of short-term goals?

_____

_____

_____

Activity F *Use the clues to complete the crossword puzzle.*

Across

1. The first step of the nursing process
2. Expected or desired outcome
3. Type of assessment; information that provides more details about specific problems and expands the original data base
4. Data consisting of information that only the client feels and can describe

Down

5. Objective data
6. Last step of the nursing process

SECTION III: APPLYING YOUR KNOWLEDGE

Activity G *During assessment, the nurse collects information to determine areas of abnormal function, risk factors that contribute to health problems, and client strengths. Read the scenario and answer the questions that follow.*

A client reports to the emergency room with chest pain. The medical file shows that the client has a history of hospitalization for chest pain. The family members inform the nurse that the client is a chain smoker. The nurse performs an initial assessment to plan the care.

1. What are the sources of data in this case?

   _____

   _____

   _____

2. What types of assessment data should be obtained in this case? Group them into subjective and objective data.

   _____

   _____

   _____

SECTION IV: PRACTICING FOR NCLEX

Activity H *Answer the following questions.*

1. A client is admitted to a health care facility with cramping pain in the abdomen. The nurse interviews the client, performs the initial assessment, and records the vital signs. Which of the following data collected by the nurse can be classified as objective data?

   a. Pain in the abdomen
   b. High blood pressure
   c. Tingling sensation
   d. Itching in the nose

2. A client with Cushing's disease is admitted after falling on the road. He has an open leg wound. Which of the following nursing diagnoses should be given the highest priority?

   a. Risk for infection
   b. Impaired physical mobility

   c. Disturbed body image
   d. Risk for delayed recovery

3. When caring for a client who has had a stroke, which of the following actions should the nurse perform first?

   a. Implement nursing care
   b. Plan nursing action
   c. Perform physical assessment
   d. Ascertain nursing goals

4. The following nursing diagnosis is entered in the client's plan of care. Which one of these diagnoses would be of least priority?

   a. Altered breathing pattern
   b. Ineffective coping
   c. Altered elimination needs
   d. Risk for body image disturbance

5. A nurse is caring for a client who receives anticoagulant therapy after mitral valve replacement. The nurse understands that the nursing diagnosis of highest priority would be

   a. Risk for physical injury
   b. Risk for infection
   c. Risk for imbalanced fluid volume
   d. Ineffective health maintenance

6. A nurse is giving post-operative care to a client after total hip replacement. Which of the following are short-term goals for this client?

   a. To ambulate the client to a bedside chair
   b. To help the client return to activities of daily life
   c. To maintain a healthy and active lifestyle
   d. To prevent repeat surgery in the client

7. A client is admitted to the health care center with profuse, watery stools. The client informs the nurse that he had eaten out the previous evening with family and friends, and had rich food because he did not want to be different from his peers. The client has a history of ulcerative colitis and is restricted from having fat-rich food. Which of the following nursing diagnoses is the most appropriate for such a client?

   a. Risk for body image disturbance
   b. Risk for situational self-esteem
   c. Ineffective health maintenance
   d. Risk for impaired nutritional intake

8. A client complains of pain in the right flank. Which of the following data gathered from the client are objective data?

a. Pricking pain in the flank

b. Grade 2 pain on the pain scale

c. Dull, throbbing pain

d. Cramping pain in the flank

9. A client is brought to the post-operative room after surgery for disc prolapse. Which of the following is a long-term goal for the client?

a. To prevent infection at the surgical site

b. To avoid putting strain on the back during the immediate post-operative period

c. To prevent recurrence by practicing body mechanics

d. To ambulate and perform activities of daily life

10. A nurse is assessing a client with renal calculus. The client received one shot of analgesic 2 hours earlier. The client is scared that the pain will come back, noting that it was the worst pain he had ever experienced. Taking into account the client's concerns, which of the following nursing diagnoses would be appropriate?

a. Impaired coping mechanism related to severe pain

b. Anxiety related to anticipation of recurrent severe pain

c. Pain related to presence of calculus in the kidney

d. Impaired elimination resulting from obstruction of urinary tract

11. Which of the following are the potential nursing diagnoses for a comatose client?

a. Risk for disuse syndrome

b. Ineffective breathing pattern

c. Impaired physical mobility

d. Total self-care deficit

12. A pregnant woman in her third trimester is admitted with spotting. She is tense and continuously inquires about the safety of her baby. Which of the following nursing diagnoses is the most appropriate for the client?

a. Risk for deficient fluid volume

b. Fear related to unpredictable outcome

c. Activity intolerance as a result of pregnancy

d. Risk for impaired urinary elimination

13. A nurse is caring for a diabetic client who has a wound. Which of the following components of the nursing care plan should be performed first?

a. To change the dressing of the wound

b. To arrange articles for dressing

c. To assess the condition of the wound

d. To record the findings of the wound

14. A nurse is planning care for a client who is receiving nasogastric feeds. Which of the following nursing diagnoses should the nurse identify as the highest priority?

a. Altered bowel elimination

b. Risk for imbalanced fluid volume

c. Risk for imbalanced nutrition

d. Risk for lung aspiration

15. A client is brought to the emergency room with a head injury. After an initial assessment, the client is taken to the operating room for removal of a blood clot. Which of the following would be part of the focus assessments for the client? Select all that apply.

a. Conducting postoperative surgical assessments

b. Conducting urine analysis on admission

c. Monitoring pain before and after administering medications

d. Checking the neurologic status of a client with a head injury

e. Inquiring about the dietary habits of the client

16. A client with a spinal cord injury is paralyzed from his neck down. The client frequently picks a fight with fellow patients on petty issues and often complains about the nursing staff. The nurse interprets that the client is inappropriately using the defense mechanism of displacement. Which of the following would be an appropriate nursing diagnosis for the client?

a. Risk for disuse syndrome

b. Deficient diversional activity

c. Ineffective coping

d. Disturbed self-esteem

17. A nurse is caring for a patient on hormone therapy. The client has a nursing diagnosis of disturbed body image related to alopecia. Which of the following plans should be implemented, relating to the nursing diagnosis?

a. Teach the client about use of wigs

b. Teach the client about use of cosmetics

c. Teach the client to use mild shampoo

d. Teach the client the method to wash the hair and scalp

18. A client reports to the health care center with complaints of diarrhea and vomiting after having pizza at a party. The nurse conducts an interview and collects the following assessment data. Which of the following data are considered subjective data? Select all that apply.

a. High temperature

b. Pain in abdomen

c. Tenesmus

d. Nausea

e. High blood pressure

CHAPTER 3

Laws and Ethics

SECTION I: LEARNING OBJECTIVES

- Name six types of laws.
- Discuss the purpose of nurse practice acts and the role of the state board of nursing.
- Explain the difference between intentional and unintentional torts.
- Describe the difference between negligence and malpractice.
- Identify three reasons a nurse should obtain professional liability insurance.
- List five ways that a nurse's professional liability can be mitigated in the case of a lawsuit.
- Define the term *ethics*.
- Explain the purpose for a code of ethics.
- Describe two types of ethical theories.
- Name and explain six ethical principles that apply to health care.
- List five ethical issues common in nursing practice.

SECTION II: ASSESSING YOUR UNDERSTANDING

Activity A *Fill in the blanks.*

1. _____ laws are enacted by federal, state, or local legislatures.

2. _____ means the duty to be honest and to avoid deceiving or misleading a client.

3. _____ is ethical study based on duty or moral obligations.

4. _____ insurance is a contract between a person or corporation and a company willing to provide legal services and financial assistance when the policyholder is involved in a malpractice lawsuit; it is necessary for all nurses.

5. _____ is an unlawful act in which untrue information harms a person's reputation.

6. _____ is a litigation in which one person asserts that a physical, emotional, or financial injury was a consequence of another person's actions or failure to act.

7. _____, also known as *utilitarianism*, is ethical theory based on final outcomes.

8. A(n)_____ is a serious criminal offense, such as murder, falsifying medical records, insurance fraud, and stealing narcotics.

9. _____ law is also known as judicial law.

10. _____ laws are legal provisions through which federal, state, and local agencies maintain self-regulation.

Activity B *Consider the following figure.*

```
┌─────────────────────────────────────────────────────────────────────────────┐
│ THREE RIVERS AREA HOSPITAL INCIDENT REPORT            Addressograph           │
│ Confidential - DO NOT DUPLICATE                                               │
│ Forward to Risk Management within 48 hours                                    │
│ Identification  Sex  Age  Incident Date  Time   Shift   Department            │
│ _Inpatient    _M _  _/_/_     :    _1st                                       │
│ _Outpatient   _F                   _2nd   _____                            │
│ _Visitor                           _3rd                                       │
│ ═══════════════════════════════════════════════════════════════════════════ │
│ Reason for hospitalization/presence on premises: _____ │
│                                                                               │
│ I.   Location of Incident           II.  Type of Incident                     │
│      _Patient Room #_____               _Fall              _Treatment/Procedure │
│      _Patient Bathroom                   _Medication        _Equipment         │
│      _Corridor                           _Infusion          _Needle/Sponge Count │
│      _Other _____             _Lost/Found        _Other_____   │
│                                          _Burn                                 │
│ III. Description of Incident _____ │
│      _____ │
│      _____ │
│ IV.  Nature of Incident                                                       │
│      A.  Falls:                                                               │
│      Activity Order:    Pt. Condition Prior to:  Fall Involved:   Patient/Visitor was: │
│      _Restraints        _Weak, unsteady          _Chair, W/C      _Lying       │
│      _Bedrest only      _Alert, oriented         _Stretcher       _Standing    │
│      _BRP               _Disoriented/confused    _Tub/Shower      _Getting on/off │
│      _Up w/asst.        _Senile                  _Toilet          _Sitting     │
│      _Up AD LIB         _Unconscious             _Floor Condition(below) _Ambulating │
│                         _Medicated/Sedated       _Bed            _Other_____ │
│                         Med. Name _____        _Side Rails Up   _____  │
│                         Last Dose _____        _Side Rails Down              │
│      B.  Medications:                                                          │
│      Incident Involved:                          Factors:                      │
│      _Wrong Med, Tx, Procedure  _Adverse Reaction  _Patient I.D. Not Checked   │
│      _Wrong Patient             _Infiltration      _Transcription              │
│      _Wrong Time                _Other_____     _Labeling                   │
│      _Omission                  _____        _Physician orders not clear │
│      _Incorrect Dose            _____        _Physician orders not checked │
│      _Incorrect Method of       _____        _Misread label/dose         │
│       Administration                               _Charting                   │
│                                                    _Wrong Med from Pharmacy    │
│                                                    _Defective equipment        │
│                                                    _Communications             │
│                                                    _Other_____              │
│      C.  Other:                                                               │
│      _Loss of Property          _Equipment malfunction  _Patient ID            │
│      _Struck by object, equipment _Anesthesia           _Other_____         │
│ V.   Nature of Injury (Injury sustained as a result of incident):             │
│      _Asphyxia, Strangulation,  _Fracture or dislocation _Burn or Scald        │
│       Inhalation                _Viscera Injury          _Chemical Burn        │
│      _Head Injury               _Sprain or strain        _No injury            │
│      _Contagious or infectious  _Contusion, Cut,         _No apparent injury   │
│       Disease Exposure           Laceration              _Other_____        │
│ VI.  Action Taken:                                                            │
│      Physician  _Yes    PT/Visitor seen by MD/T&EC    MD Name                  │
│      Notified   _No     _Yes      _No       _____ Time  :   │
│      Physician's Findings: _____ │
│                                                                               │
│      Other follow up:  _No  _Yes - Specify_____  │
│                                                                               │
│      _____  _/_/_      _____  _/_/_                      │
│      Name of Person Reporting  Date   Department Director  Date                │
│                                                                               │
│      _____  _/_/_      _____  _/_/_                      │
│      Supervisor           Date    Risk Management     Date       8311-109      │
└─────────────────────────────────────────────────────────────────────────────┘
```

1. Identify the figure.

_____

_____

2. What is the role of nurse in filling out an incident report?

_____

_____

3. What are the important factors the nurse should keep in mind while completing an incident report?

_____

_____

LIVING WILL

TO: My family, physicians and all those concerned with my care

I, _____, the undersigned "principal", presently residing at _____, _____, and being an adult of sound mind, make this declaration as a directive to be followed if for any reason I become unable to make or communicate decisions regarding my medical care.

I do not want medical treatment that will keep me alive if I am unconscious and there is no reasonable prospect that I will ever be conscious again (even if I am not going to die soon in my medical condition) or if I am near death from an illness or injury with no reasonable prospect of recovery. The procedures and treatment to be withheld and withdrawn include, without limitation, surgery, antibiotics, cardiac and pulmonary resuscitation, respiratory support, and artificially administered feeding and fluids. I direct that treatment be limited to measures to keep me comfortable and to relieve pain, even if such measures shorten my life.

[OPTIONAL] I wish to live out my last days at home rather than in a hospital, if it does not jeopardize the chance of my recovery to a meaningful and conscious life and does not impose an undue burden on my family.

[OPTIONAL] If, upon my death, any of my tissue or organs would be of value for transplantation, therapy, advancement of medical or dental science, research, or other medical, educational or scientific purpose, I freely give my permission to the donation of such tissue or organs.

These directions are the exercise of my legal right to refuse treatment. Therefore, I expect my family, physicians, health care facilities and all concerned with my care to regard themselves as legally and morally bound to act in accordance with my wishes, and in so doing to be free from any liability for having followed my directions.

IN WITNESS WHEREOF, I have executed this declaration, as my free and voluntary act and deed, this _____ day of _____, 2003.

_____   _____
Principal's name: WITNESS:

4. Identify the figure.

_____

_____

_____

5. What is meant by advance directives?

_____

_____

_____

6. Can the nurse sign as a witness in a living will?

_____

_____

_____

Activity C *Match the legal terms in column A with their description in column B.*

Column A

_____ **1.** Assault

_____ **2.** Battery

_____ **3.** Slander

_____ **4.** Libel

Column B

A. Damaging statements written and read by others

B. An act in which bodily harm is threatened or attempted

C. Unauthorized physical contact that includes touching a person's body, clothing, chair, or bed

D. Character attack uttered orally in the presence of others

Activity D *Briefly answer the following.*

1. What is meant by allocation of scarce resources?

_____

_____

_____

2. What is meant by code status?

_____

_____

_____

3. What is a living will?

_____

_____

_____

4. What are some common ethical issues that recur in nursing practices?

_____

_____

_____

5. What is autonomy in client care?

_____

_____

_____

Activity E *Use the clues to complete the crossword puzzle.*

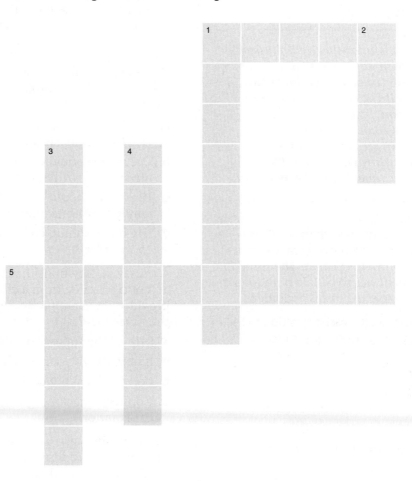

Across

1. Statutes that protect personal freedoms and rights
5. Devices or chemicals that restrict movement

Down

1. Laws used to prosecute those who commit crimes
2. Rules of conduct established and enforced by the government
3. Being faithful to work-related commitments and obligations
4. Unauthorized physical contact

SECTION III: APPLYING YOUR KNOWLEDGE

Activity F *Battery is unauthorized physical contact that can include touching a person's body, clothing, chair, or bed. A plaintiff can claim battery even if the contact causes no actual physical harm. The criterion is that contact happened without the plaintiff's consent. Nurses have great responsibility to avoid lawsuits regarding client care. Please answer the following questions in this regard.*

A client is brought to the emergency department with blunt injury on the abdomen resulting from a motor vehicle accident. The client is unconscious and not accompanied by his family, but has his identification in his pocket. The surgeon decides that the client has to be taken up for surgery, because he is bleeding in his abdomen.

1. What should the health care team do in case there is nobody to provide consent for surgery?

   _____

   _____

   _____

2. Should the act be considered battery?

   _____

   _____

   _____

SECTION IV: PRACTICING FOR NCLEX

Activity G *Answer the following questions.*

1. A client is experiencing chest pain and asks to see the physician. The nurse calls upon the physician, who is busy. When the physician visits the client, the nurse overhears him telling the client that the nurse is very inefficient. Which of the following legal provisions could the physician be charged with?
   a. Tort
   b. Assault
   c. Slander
   d. Libel

2. A physician asks the nurse to remove the nasogastric tube from a client who has been in a coma for the past few months. The physician informs the nurse that the family members had requested him to do so. What should be the first action of the nurse with regard to the legal implication of removing the feeding tube?
   a. The nurse should carry out the order as told by the physician
   b. The nurse should check the records for the physician's written order
   c. The nurse should check the records for the family's authorization
   d. The nurse should check the records for the court order

3. A nurse on duty finds that her colleague is accepting money from a client for the care provided. What appropriate action should the nurse take?
   a. Inform the supervisor about the incident
   b. Ignore the incident and keep silent
   c. Call the local police to the nursing unit
   d. Confront the colleague and ask for an explanation

4. A client is brought to the emergency department with a head injury sustained from a motor vehicle accident. The surgeon determines that the client needs to undergo immediate surgery for the removal of a clot to save his life. The client is not accompanied by any family member. Which of the following action should be a priority?
   a. Contact the client's family and wait for them to give consent for surgery
   b. Get the client operated on, assuming that the consent is implied
   c. Sign the consent form yourself and later explain to the family
   d. Inform the supervisor and request that she sign the consent form

5. A well-known personality has been admitted to the health care facility with chest pain. A person approaches the nurse posing as the client's family member and asks about the client's health details. The nurse reveals the medical details about the client. Later, it is discovered that this person was a press reporter and not a family member. Which legal provision has the nurse violated?

   a. Right to information

   b. Breach of nursing duty

   c. Client's right to privacy

   d. Defamation of the client

6. A physician on a client visit tells the nurse to increase the insulin dose to 10 units. He requests the nurse to write down the orders on his behalf, because he has to rush to the intensive care unit (ICU). What should be the nurse's response in this case?

   a. Tell the physician to come back and write the orders

   b. Carry out the instruction without a written order

   c. Write the order on behalf of the physician

   d. Inform the client about the change in drug dosage

7. While administering regular insulin shots to a client, the nurse notices that the client is sweating profusely. Assuming that the sweating is a result of the warm weather, the nurse ignores the client's condition. Later, the client is found unconscious resulting from hypoglycemia. Which of the following legal terms appropriately describe the nurse's action?

   a. Defamation

   b. Negligence

   c. Battery

   d. Assault

8. A nurse is caring for a client who has terminal cancer. The client states that his lawyer would be coming to prepare his living will and requests her to sign as a witness. What should the nurse's action be?

   a. Willingly signing as a witness to the living will

   b. Calling the physician to sign as a witness

   c. Politely informing the client that she is not authorized to sign

   d. Calling the nurse supervisor to sign as a witness

9. A nurse enters the client's room and finds that the plug point for the cardiac monitor has a short circuit. The nurse turns off the main switch and calls for the electrician. The nurse assesses whether the client has sustained any injury, makes him comfortable, and proceeds to fill in the incident report. What should the nurse's next action be?

   a. Informing the physician and nurse supervisor about the incident

   b. Making a copy of the incident report to give to the physician

   c. Making a copy of the incident report and putting it in the client's record

   d. Making a note in the client's record about the incident report

10. A client who has undergone arthroscopy is advised to ambulate only with assistance. The nurse finds that the client is trying to walk without any support and warns him that he may fall and hurt himself. Later the client loses his balance and falls down, sustaining an injury to the forehead. Which of the following would provide the nurse immunity from a possible lawsuit?

   a. Good Samaritan Law

   b. Assumption of risk

   c. Statute of limitation

   d. Judicial law

11. Which of the following situations is an example of assault that a nurse may experience when performing her nursing duties?

   a. A nurse telling the client he cannot leave the health care facility

   b. A nurse restraining a client from being discharged without physician consent

   c. A nurse threatening to turn off the signal system of communication

   d. A nurse discussing confidential client information with a friend

12. A client who is scheduled for barium ingestion tests receives a food tray at mealtime. The client refuses to eat the food because the physician had instructed him not to take anything orally. The nurse insists that it is not necessary to be fasting before a barium investigation. The client takes dinner and, as a result, cannot undergo the barium ingestion test. The determination of negligence in this situation is based on which of the following factors?

a. The dietary department sent a meal for the client

b. Harm resulted because the nurse did not act reasonably

c. The nurse did not confirm the order with the physician

d. The nurse insisted that the patient have the meal

13. A client feels that he is not getting appropriate treatment and wants to leave the hospital. He informs his caregiver of this. On realizing that the client is leaving without proper discharge, the nurse tries to stop the client by restraining him. What legal charges could be put on the nurse for her action? Select all that apply.

a. Assault

b. Battery

c. Slander

d. False imprisonment

e. Libel

14. A nurse has published a research report on human immunodeficiency virus (HIV). A client finds that his name is mentioned in the report, along with the fact that the client had contracted the infection from a prostitute. Which of the following legal provisions apply to the nurse? Select all that apply.

a. Felony

b. Invasion of privacy

c. Libel

d. Slander

e. Misdemeanor

15. A client is experiencing psychotic symptoms and is becoming violent. The nurse determines that the client needs to be restrained because he can be potentially harmful. Which of the following are appropriate nursing actions? Select all that apply.

a. The nurse should sedate the client and then restrain him

b. The nurse should take orders from the physician for restraining

c. The nurse should document the type and duration of restraint

d. The nurse should make her own decision and restrain the client

e. The nurse should explain to the family the reason for restraining

CHAPTER 4

Health and Illness

SECTION I: LEARNING OBJECTIVES

- Describe how the World Health Organization (WHO) defines health.
- Discuss the difference between values and beliefs.
- List three health beliefs common among Americans.
- Explain the concept of holism.
- Identify five levels of human needs.
- Define illness.
- Explain the meaning of the following terms used to describe illnesses: morbidity, mortality, acute, chronic, terminal, primary, secondary, remission, exacerbation, hereditary, congenital, and idiopathic.
- Differentiate among primary, secondary, tertiary, and extended care.
- Name two programs that help finance health care for the elderly, disabled, and poor.
- List four methods to control escalating health care costs.
- Identify two national health goals targeted for the year 2010.
- Discuss five patterns that nurses use to administer client care.

SECTION II: ASSESSING YOUR UNDERSTANDING

Activity A *Fill in the blanks.*

1. Abraham Maslow is a(n) _____ who identified five levels of human needs.

2. The sum of physical, emotional, social, and spiritual health is called _____.

3. _____ denotes the number of people who died from a particular disease or condition.

4. The disorder acquired from the genetic codes of one or both parents is called a(n) _____ condition.

5. Health services provided by the first health care professional or agency a person contacts is called _____ care.

6. WHO defines health as a state of complete physical, mental, and social well-being, not merely the absence of disease or _____.

7. _____ refers to incidence of a specific disease, disorder, or injury and the rate or numbers of people affected.

8. A(n) _____ illness is a disorder that develops from a preexisting condition.

9. _____ is a federal program that finances health care costs of persons 65 years and older.

10. The nursing care pattern in which nursing personnel divide clients into groups and complete their care together is called _____ nursing.

Activity B *Consider the following figures.*

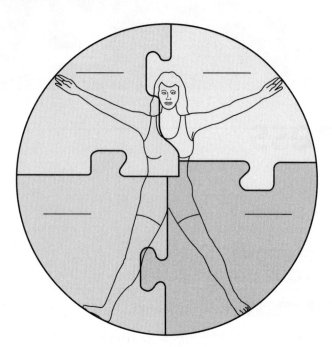

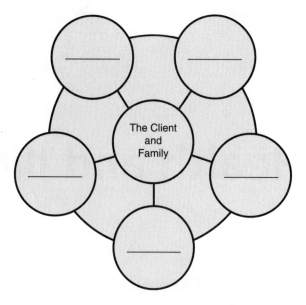

1. Identify and label the figure.

_____

_____

_____

2. List the various aspects of holism.

_____

_____

_____

3. How are the various aspects related to each other?

_____

_____

_____

4. Label the figure to indicate members of the nursing team.

_____

_____

_____

5. What is the main purpose of the nursing team?

_____

_____

_____

Activity C *Match the types of illness in column A with their descriptions in column B.*

Column A

____ **1.** Primary illness

____ **2.** Acute illness

____ **3.** Terminal illness

____ **4.** Chronic illness

Column B

A. Illness that comes on slowly and lasts a long time

B. Illness that develops independently of any other disease

C. Illness that comes on suddenly and lasts a short time

D. Illness for which there is no potential for cure

Activity D *The following are the five levels of human needs in random order as identified by Maslow's hierarchy. Write the correct sequence in the boxes provided.*

1. Physiological needs

2. Esteem and self-esteem

3. Safety and security

4. Love and belonging

5. Self-actualization

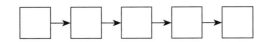

The following are some of the agencies and institutions, in random order, where people seek treatment for health problems or assistance with maintaining or promoting their health. Write the correct sequence in which health care is obtained, in the boxes provided.

1. Physiotherapy center

2. Family physician

3. Multispecialty hospital

4. Diagnostic center

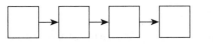

Activity E *Briefly answer the following.*

1. Why is the first level of Maslow's hierarchy of human needs very important?

_____

_____

_____

2. What are the types of illness based on duration?

_____

_____

_____

3. What are managed care organizations?

_____

_____

_____

4. What is capitation?

_____

_____

_____

5. What is nurse-managed care?

_____

_____

_____

Activity F *Use the clues to complete the crossword puzzle.*

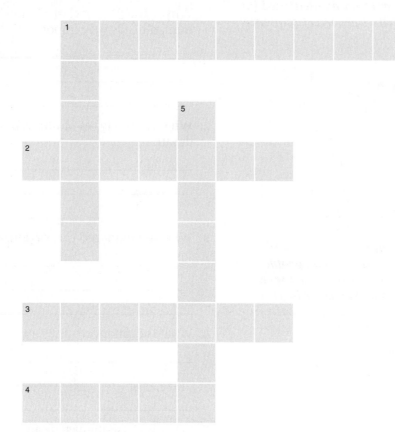

Across

1. The number of people who died from a particular disease or condition
2. A state of discomfort
3. Illness that develops independently of any other disease
4. Illness that comes on suddenly and lasts a short time

Down

1. The psychologist who identified five levels of human needs
5. A federal program that finances health care costs of persons 65 years and older

SECTION III: APPLYING YOUR KNOWLEDGE

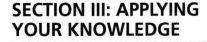 *Nursing care is based on five common management patterns: functional nursing, case method, team nursing, primary nursing, and nurse-managed care. Nurse-managed care involves a clinical pathway and typically is used in a managed care approach. Answer the following questions, which involve the nurse's role as a nurse manager.*

A client is admitted to the nursing unit for a hernioplasty. The nursing unit follows the nurse-managed care pattern of nursing care.

1. What are the responsibilities of a nurse manager?

   _____

   _____

   _____

2. What are the advantages of the nurse-managed care pattern?

   _____

   _____

   _____

SECTION IV: PRACTICING FOR NCLEX

Activity H *Answer the following questions.*

1. A client has undergone amputation of the left leg. The wound has healed well with no complications. The client will need a prosthesis to enable him to walk. The nurse understands that the client would require
   a. Primary care of a general physician
   b. Secondary care of a reconstructive surgeon
   c. Tertiary care of a sophisticated hospital
   d. Extended care of a rehabilitation center

2. A client is depressed after the death of her spouse. She does not want to meet her friends or other family members. The client has low self-esteem, because she was dependent on her spouse. Which aspect of this client's health requires immediate attention?
   a. Inability to cope
   b. Depression
   c. Low self-esteem
   d. Dependency

3. An LPN is caring for an elderly client recently diagnosed with osteoarthritis. The client informs the nurse that he has been experiencing pain in the knees for the past 4 months. The nurse understands that osteoarthritis has a
   a. Gradual onset
   b. Genetic predisposition
   c. Short disease course
   d. Short treatment regimen

4. The nurse understands that secondary illness is a disorder that develops from a preexisting condition. Which of the following is a secondary disorder?
   a. Lung disease resulting from smoking
   b. Smoking because of social causes
   c. Heart disease resulting from a damaged lung
   d. Heart disease resulting from fetal abnormalities

5. An LPN understands that remission is the disappearance of signs and symptoms associated with a particular disease. He is aware that although remission resembles a cured state, the relief may be only temporary. Which of the following disease conditions has a remission state?
   a. Gout
   b. Heart attack
   c. Common cold
   d. Varicose veins

6. A student nurse in her clinical rotation is posted to a new nursing unit. She observes that the nursing staff follows the functional nursing approach of nursing model. The nurse understands that functional nursing is a nursing model wherein

   a. The nursing staff is headed by a team leader

   b. The nurse manager plans the nursing care of clients

   c. One nurse plans and provides individualized nursing care

   d. A head nurse assigns specific tasks to other members

7. A nurse manager plans the nursing care of clients based on their type of case or medical diagnosis. The nurse evaluates whether predictable outcomes are met on a daily basis. The nurse manager is an important person in

   a. Team nursing

   b. Functional nursing

   c. Nurse-managed care

   d. Case method

8. The LPN understands that managed care organizations are private insurers and agencies that provide health care services. Federal policies like Medicare and Medicaid also exist for people who cannot afford services of managed care organizations. Which of the following statements is an important component of Medicare?

   a. They bargain with providers for quality care at reasonable costs

   b. They reimburse hospital charges based on the diagnostic-related group

   c. They provide client education to decrease the risk of disease

   d. They monitor and manage fiscal and client outcomes

9. An LPN is caring for a client with hemophilia. The nurse understands that it is a hereditary disorder. Which of the following are hereditary disorders?

   a. Atrial septal defect

   b. Myositis

   c. Cystic fibrosis

   d. Macular edema

10. A baby is born with multiple fingers, or polydactyly. The nurse explains to the mother that it is a congenital disorder. Which of the following statements from the mother indicates the need for further education on the subject?

    a. It is the result of an abnormality in genes

    b. It is the result of faulty embryonic development

    c. It is the result of maternal exposure to infections

    d. It is the result of maternal exposure to certain drugs

11. Mortality and morbidity are measures of disease burden relating to specific diseases or conditions. Which of the following statements indicate neonatal mortality rate?

    a. Number of neonatal deaths per 1,000 deliveries

    b. Number of neonatal deaths before 1 year of age

    c. Number of neonatal deaths per 1,000 live births

    d. Number of neonatal deaths per year

12. A 50-year-old client who underwent surgery for prolapsed disc is to undergo physiotherapy after discharge. The nurse understands that a physiotherapy center is an example of

    a. Continuity of care

    b. Extended care

    c. Secondary care

    d. Tertiary care

13. In a nursing unit, the nurse delegates specific tasks to the team members and tells them to report on the completion of the task. The nurse assigns the task, supervises, and obtains feedback. Which type of nursing care is being implemented?

    a. Team nursing

    b. Functional nursing

    c. Primary nursing

    d. Nurse-managed care

14. A client admitted for arthroscopy is discharged 2 days earlier than the estimated time because he has had a fast recovery and is doing well. The client is insured through a capitation scheme. In the event of early discharge of the client, who makes the monetary benefit?

    a. The client

    b. The hospital

    c. The provider

    d. The government

15. A client presents to a family physician with symptoms of chest pain. After initial examination, the physician refers the client to a medical specialist. This is an example of

    a. Extended care

    b. Continuity of care

    c. Secondary care

    d. Primary care

16. Which of the following statements indicate a measure of mortality?

    a. Lung cancer accounts for 1% of all cigarette smoking-attributable illnesses

    b. Each year, 440,000 people die of a cigarette smoking-attributable illness

    c. Cigarette smoking results in 5.6 million potential lives lost each year

    d. Seventy-five billion dollars is lost in the direct medical costs of smoking-attributable illnesses

17. Assessment of a client with minor burns on the face and hands reveals the following main findings. Place the needs in order of priority of nursing care.

    a. Inability to perform daily activities

    b. Pain in the open wound

    c. Anxiety and apprehension about the treatment

    d. Inability to interact with friends and family

18. A nurse is caring for several clients in a health care facility. Which among the following cases are acute disorders? Select all that apply.

    a. Diabetes mellitus

    b. Influenza

    c. Measles

    d. Hypertension

    e. Conjunctivitis

19. Team nursing is a pattern in which nursing personnel divide the clients into groups and complete their care together. What is the responsibility of the team leader?

    a. To care for clients who are confined to bed

    b. To administer medicines and injections

    c. To assign, supervise, and evaluate care

    d. To act as a liaison with other departments for client care

20. The nurse understands that there are five common management patterns. Each has advantages and disadvantages. Which of the following patterns has a conference as its most important component?

    a. Functional nursing

    b. Case method

    c. Team nursing

    d. Nurse-managed care

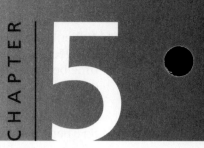

CHAPTER 5

Homeostasis, Adaptation, and Stress

SECTION I: LEARNING OBJECTIVES

- Explain homeostasis.
- List four categories of stressors that affect homeostasis.
- Identify two beliefs about the body and mind based on the concept of holism.
- Identify the purpose of adaptation and two possible outcomes of unsuccessful adaptation.
- Trace the structures through which adaptive changes take place.
- Differentiate between sympathetic and parasympathetic adaptive responses.
- Define stress.
- List 10 factors that affect the stress response.
- Discuss the three stages and consequences of the general adaptation syndrome.
- Name three levels of prevention that apply to the reduction or management of stress-related disorders.
- Explain psychological adaptation and two possible outcomes.
- List eight nursing activities helpful to the care of clients prone to stress.
- List four approaches for preventing, reducing, or eliminating a stress response.

SECTION II: ASSESSING YOUR UNDERSTANDING

Activity A *Fill in the blanks.*

1. _____ are chemical messengers synthesized in the neurons.

2. Neurotransmitters, when released, temporarily bind to receptor sites on the _____ neuron and transmit their information.

3. Another chemical messenger, called a(n) _____, is a separate type of neurotransmitter.

4. _____ stabilizes mood, induces sleep, and regulates temperature.

5. The neurotransmitter _____ heightens arousal and increases energy.

6. The central nervous system is composed of the brain and _____.

7. The _____ enables people to think abstractly and helps in accumulating and storing memories.

8. The _____ is responsible for regulating and maintaining blood pressure.

9. The pituitary gland is connected to the _____ through both vascular connections and nerve endings.

10. The _____ gland in the brain is known as the master gland.

Activity B *Consider the following figure.*

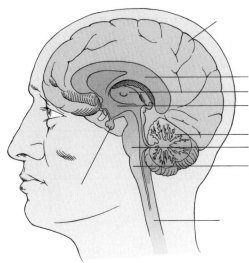

1. Identify and label the figure.

_____

_____

_____

2. What is the function of each component?

_____

_____

_____

Activity C *Match the physiologic stress response in column A with its corresponding characteristics in column B.*

Column A

___ **1.** Alarm stage

___ **2.** Stage of resistance

___ **3.** Stage of exhaustion

Column B

A. Adaptation/resistance can no longer protect the person experiencing the stressor

B. Prepares the person for a "fight-or-flight" response

C. Returns the person experiencing the stressor to the stage of normalcy

Activity D *Presented here, in random order, are stress-related responses. Write the correct sequence in the boxes provided below.*

1. Adrenal glands secrete additional norepinephrine and epinephrine.

2. Storage vesicles release norepinephrine.

3. The body might return to the homeostasis stage.

4. The adrenal cortex releases cortisol, a stress hormone.

5. The person is at a risk of severe infections or cancer.

6. The person is prepared for a fight-or-flight response.

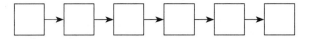

Presented here, in random order, are steps for nurses to follow while treating a stressed client. Write the correct sequence in the boxes provided below.

1. Eliminate or reduce the stressors.

2. Identify the stressors.

3. Prevent additional stressors.

4. Assess the client's response to stress.

5. Implement stress reduction and stress management techniques.

6. Promote the client's physiologic adaptive responses.

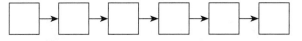

Activity E *Briefly answer the following.*

1. What is the difference between the sympathetic and the parasympathetic nervous systems?

_____

_____

_____

2. Define feedback loop.

_____

_____

_____

3. What is the scientific definition of stress?

_____

_____

_____

4. Briefly describe the three stages of stress.

_____

_____

_____

5. What are coping strategies? List the types of coping strategies.

_____

_____

_____

6. How can you help prevent or minimize stress-related illnesses?

_____

_____

_____

Activity F *Use the clues to complete the crossword puzzle.*

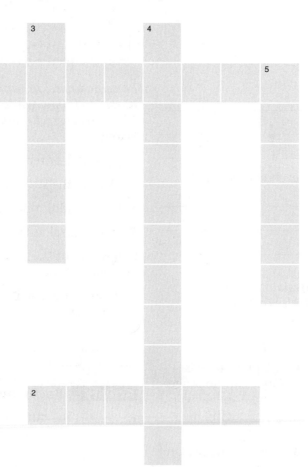

Across

1. Chemicals manufactured in the body
2. The first stage of stress response

Down

3. Enables people to think abstractly, and use and understand language
4. This means staying the same
5. Physiologic and behavioral responses to disequilibrium

SECTION III: APPLYING YOUR KNOWLEDGE

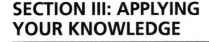 *Stress is a physiologic and behavioral response to disequilibrium. It has physical, emotional, and cognitive effects. Although all humans have the capacity to adapt to stress, not everyone responds to similar stressors exactly the same. Read the scenario and answer the questions that follow, which involve the nurse's role in caring for the client with stress.*

A 50-year-old client with a high glucose level is undergoing stress-related treatment. The client seems to be getting aggressive. The nurse stands in front of the client and says, "Tell me about the incident that is disturbing you." The client, who is seated, seems disturbed and is sweating profusely. The nurse repeats the instructions, but the client becomes agitated and does not respond to the nurse.

1. What measures could the nurse take to ensure an accurate assessment of the client's condition?

   _____

   _____

   _____

2. What care should the nurse take during further discussions and care of the client?

   _____

   _____

   _____

SECTION IV: PRACTICING FOR NCLEX

Activity H *Answer the following questions.*

1. A client with a family history of hypertension and high blood pressure visits the health care facility for a physical examination. As a primary level of stress prevention, what should the nurse do?

   a. Regularly monitor the client's blood pressure

   b. Teach principles to maintaining blood pressure

   c. Prescribe medicines for hypertension

   d. Prescribe a strict diet and exercise routine

2. A client who had been involved in a minor car accident is stressed about the cost of recovery. Under the nurse's guidance, the client starts focusing on the positive aspect of being physically unharmed. Which of the following techniques is the nurse implementing?

   a. Alternative thinking

   b. Alternative behavior

   c. Alternative lifestyle

   d. Adaptive activities

3. The nurse is caring for a client with a family history of hypertension. As a secondary level of stress prevention, what should the nurse do?

   a. Regularly monitor the client's blood pressure

   b. Teach principles to maintain the blood pressure

   c. Prescribe medicines for hypertension

   d. Prescribe a strict diet and exercise routine

4. A client visits the medical center with complaints of stress. He had lost his left arm in an accident and has been complaining that his family has not been treating him properly since the accident. He feels he has become a burden to his family. What should be the nurse's observation in this case?

   a. The client is resorting to non-therapeutic coping strategies

   b. The client is adopting therapeutic coping strategies

   c. The client is using coping mechanisms to deal with his situation

   d. The client is suffering from stress-related disorders

5. A client diagnosed with stress and depression is advised by the nurse to share his frustrations with other supportive people and also to adopt an assertive approach to the situation. Which of the following stress management techniques is the nurse implementing?

   a. Alternative thinking

   b. Alternative behaviors

   c. Alternative lifestyles

   d. Adaptive activities

6. A nurse is caring for a client with insomnia. Which of the following neurotransmitters should the nurse be aware of that would help induce sleep in the client?

   a. Norepinephrine

   b. Serotonin

   c. Dopamine

   d. Endorphins

7. A client complains of pain in the arm muscles. The nurse suggests a body massage for pain relief. Identify the chemical that will be released by the massage, which will help stop the pain.

   a. Endorphins

   b. Gamma-aminobutyric acid

   c. Substance P

   d. Acetylcholine

8. A client is admitted to the clinic with high blood pressure. Upon interviewing the client, the nurse finds that she is suffering from stress at the workplace. The client is very timid in nature and is unable to refuse any work that comes from her colleagues or boss. What should the nurse advise the client?

   a. The nurse should advise that the client change her job

   b. The nurse should advise that the client accept her duties and situation

   c. The nurse should advise the client to adopt alternative behavior

   d. The nurse should advise the client to undergo therapy to reduce stress

9. A 10-year-old boy, who has gone into depression after the death of his mother, is accompanied by his father to the health care facility. The nurse performs routine tests on the boy and finds that he has very high blood pressure and his heartbeat is irregularly high. What should the nurse conclude in this case?

   a. The boy is in the exhaustion stage of stress

   b. The boy is in the alarm stage of stress

   c. The boy is in the resistance stage of stress

   d. The boy is in a state of homeostasis

10. In which of the following situations would the nurse's prescription for therapeutic intervention to a stressed client be most effective?

    a. The spouse of the client has died recently

    b. The client has lost a lot of money from gambling

    c. The client has recently lost his job

    d. The client has moved to a low-income neighborhood

11. A 55-year-old client is suffering from depression after his spouse died. The children of the client are married and settled in other states. The nurse advises him to get a pet dog to stay with him for company, and also to listen to soothing music to uplift his mood. Which of the following techniques is the nurse implementing?

    a. Alternative thinking

    b. Alternative behaviors

    c. Alternative lifestyles

    d. Adaptive activities

12. A client has been admitted to the medical center with severe depression and stress. How should the nurse attempt to treat the client?

    a. Teach the client the importance of being happy and unstressed

    b. Administer therapies that alter mood and feelings

    c. Administer antidepressants to counter stress

    d. Find the factors that have caused stress and depression

13. A client who has been facing financial distress for a long time complains of bowel infections and allergies. The client has also developed rheumatoid arthritis. The nurse feels that the immune system of the client is not strong. What should the nurse conclude?

    a. The client is in the exhaustion stage of stress

    b. The client is in the resistance stage of stress

    c. The client is in the alarm stage of stress

    d. The client is in a state of homeostasis or balance

14. The nurse is caring for a client who is admitted to the medical center with high levels of stress and anxiety. Upon questioning, the client states that his mother also suffered from stress. How should the nurse help the client? Select all that apply.

   a. Advise the client to undergo stress management therapy

   b. Advise the client to accept his duties and situation

   c. Advise the client to adopt assertive behavior at the workplace

   d. Advise the client to make changes to his home environment

   e. Advise the client to take medication to counter stress

15. A client is admitted to the medical center with a high level of stress. Order the following tasks in the most likely sequence in which the nurse should perform them while caring for this client.

   a. Prevent other factors from causing stress

   b. Analyze how the client responds to stress

   c. Identify the reasons for stress

   d. Implement stress reduction and stress management techniques

   e. Eliminate or reduce the factors causing stress

16. The nurse is caring for a client with high levels of stress. The client was involved in an accident, during which his car was severely damaged. Order the stress-related responses that occur in the client's brain in the most likely sequence in which they would have occurred.

   a. The hypothalamus releases corticotropin-releasing factor

   b. The storage vesicles within the sympathetic nervous system neurons rapidly release norepinephrine

   c. The adrenal glands secrete additional norepinephrine and epinephrine

   d. The adrenal cortex releases cortisol, a stress hormone

   e. The pituitary gland secretes adrenocorticotropic hormone

CHAPTER 6

Culture and Ethnicity

SECTION I: LEARNING OBJECTIVES

- Differentiate culture, race, and ethnicity.
- Discuss two factors that interfere with perceiving others as individuals.
- Explain why American culture is described as being Anglicized.
- List at least five characteristics of Anglo-American culture.
- Define the term *subculture* and list four major subcultures in the United States.
- List five ways in which people from subcultural groups differ from Anglo-Americans.
- Describe four characteristics of culturally sensitive care.
- List at least five ways to demonstrate cultural sensitivity.

SECTION II: ASSESSING YOUR UNDERSTANDING

Activity A *Fill in the blanks.*

1. _____ is a term used when referring to a collective group of people who differ from the dominant group in terms of cultural characteristics, such as language, and physical characteristics, such as skin color, or both.

2. African Americans and people from _____ countries lack the glucose 6-phosphate dehydrogenase (G-6-PD) enzyme.

3. _____ are unique cultural groups that coexist within the dominant culture.

4. _____ is a supposition that a person shares cultural characteristics with others of a similar background.

5. _____ is the belief that one's own ethnicity is superior to all others.

6. _____ is a digestive enzyme that converts lactose, the sugar in milk, into the simpler sugars glucose and galactose.

7. _____ medicine refers to the health practices unique to a particular group of people and has come to mean the methods of disease prevention or treatment outside mainstream conventional practice.

8. A(n) _____ is a holy man with curative powers in folk medicine.

9. Mongolian spots, an example of _____, are dark-blue areas on the lower back of darkly pigmented infants and children.

10. _____ is the ability to speak a second language.

Activity B *Consider the following figure.*

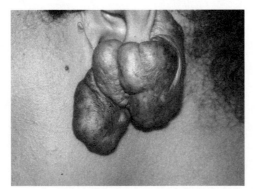

1. Identify the skin condition shown in the figure.

_____

_____

_____

2. Which skin types commonly show this condition and why?

_____

_____

_____

Activity C *Match the names of beliefs concerning illness in column A with its description in column B.*

Column A

____ **1.** Yin/yang

____ **2.** Hot/cold

____ **3.** Naturalistic

____ **4.** Magico-religious

Column B

A. Supernatural forces contribute to disease or health

B. Humans and nature must be in balance or harmony to remain healthy

C. Balanced forces promote health

D. Increasing or reducing temperature restores health

Activity D *Briefly answer the following.*

1. What is meant by culture?

_____

_____

_____

2. What are the characteristics of minority groups?

_____

_____

_____

3. What is the difference between stereotyping and generalizing?

_____

_____

_____

4. What is the current impact of ethnocentrism on different parts of the world?

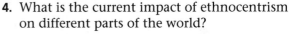

_____

_____

5. What are the various subcultures in the United States?

_____

_____

_____

Activity E *Use the clues to complete the crossword puzzle.*

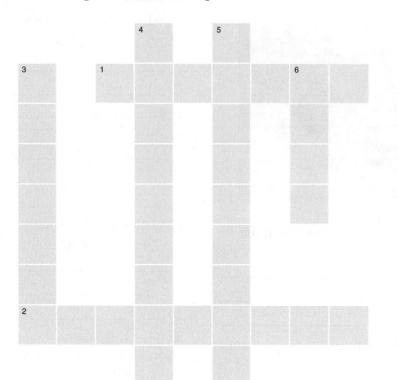

Across

1. Values, beliefs, and practices of a particular group
2. Aspect of a person's life involving religious beliefs

Down

3. People who trace their ethnic origin to Latin or South America
4. A Latino practitioner who is thought to have spiritual and medicinal powers
5. Bond or kinship a person feels with his or her country of birth or place of ancestral origin
6. Term used to categorize people with genetically shared physical characteristics

SECTION III: APPLYING YOUR KNOWLEDGE

Activity F *To provide culturally sensitive care, nurses must become skilled at managing language differences, understanding biologic and physiologic variations, promoting health teaching that will reduce prevalent diseases, and respecting alternative health beliefs or practices.*

A client who is Native American is admitted to the nursing unit for abdominoplasty. The nurse understands that behavioral patterns of Native Americans differ from one culture to another. Answer the following questions, which involve the nurse's understanding of cultural differences and their application.

1. What should the nurse keep in mind while interviewing the client?

   _____

   _____

   _____

2. How should the nurse demonstrate culturally sensitive nursing care?

   _____

   _____

   _____

SECTION IV: PRACTICING FOR NCLEX

Activity G *Answer the following questions.*

1. The nurse is interviewing a Latino client who is scheduled for a routine physical examination after chemotherapy. What actions by the nurse demonstrate cultural sensitivity?
   a. Sit far away from the client
   b. Provide information and ask questions slowly
   c. Use medical terminology during the interview
   d. Ask the client to express himself emotionally

2. The nurse is assisting an Asian American client in eating who has minor burns on his hands. The nurse is aware that Asian Americans may feel threatened with physical closeness. What would be the nurse's most appropriate action?
   a. Do not assist the client if he feels uneasy
   b. Assist the client and leave the client's room
   c. Explain to the client the purpose of the assistance
   d. Give instructions to the client regarding how to eat

3. A nurse is caring for a client with lactase deficiency. Which of the following actions should the nurse perform either to reduce or eliminate lactose?
   a. Avoid giving lactose-free milk to the client
   b. Ask the client to eat breads and cereals
   c. Avoid using foods with *pareve* on the label
   d. Ask the client to use non-dairy creamers

4. After bathing a dark-skinned client, the nurse notices that the washcloth has brown discoloration on it. What should be the reaction of the nurse in this case?
   a. Assume it is dirt and bathe the client again
   b. Consider it to be normal for the client
   c. Educate the client about personal hygiene
   d. Consider it a symptom of the disease

5. On a home visit to an African American family, the nurse finds that the 3-month-old baby has dark-blue spots on the lower back. Which of the following would be the appropriate action for the nurse to take?
   a. Inform the police of child abuse
   b. Ask the family about the spot
   c. Advise the mother to consult a doctor
   d. Consider it normal for the ethnic group

6. A client is admitted to the nursing unit with cramps, intestinal gas, and diarrhea, approximately 30 minutes after ingesting milk. Which of the following conditions should the nurse suspect the client may have?
   a. Lactase deficiency
   b. G-6-PD deficiency
   c. Antidiuretic hormone (ADH) deficiency
   d. Thyroid deficiency

7. On examining a dark-skinned client, the nurse detects the presence of keloids. What should be the nurse's reaction?

   a. Consider it pathologic
   b. Inform the physician
   c. Consider it normal
   d. Perform biochemical tests

8. A male nurse is assigned to change the dressing of a female Southeast Asian client who has an accidental wound on the knee. Keeping in mind that the people of this culture consider the female body part from the knee to the waist as private, what actions should the nurse take while dressing the wound? Select all that apply.

   a. Relieve the client's anxiety by offering an explanation
   b. Request permission from the client's husband
   c. Include a female attendant during the procedure
   d. Instruct the husband to do the procedure
   e. Allow the client's husband to stay in the room

9. A nurse is caring for an African American client who is non-cooperative with the health care team. Keeping in mind that African Americans have been victims of discrimination, what should be the nurse's actions to make the client comfortable? Select all that apply.

   a. Address the client by his or her last name
   b. Follow up thoroughly with requests
   c. Respect the client's privacy
   d. Maintain eye contact during communication
   e. Ask direct questions to the client

10. A registered nurse delegates the task of combing a client's hair to the LPN. Keeping in mind that the client is an African American woman with curly hair, what nursing actions should the LPN follow? Select all that apply.

   a. Ask the client to help you comb her hair
   b. Apply a moisturizing cream or gel
   c. Use a wide-toothed comb or pick
   d. Wet the hair with water before combing
   e. Let the client's hair remain as it is currently

The Nurse–Client Relationship

SECTION I: LEARNING OBJECTIVES

- Name four roles that nurses perform in nurse–client relationships.
- Describe the current role expectations for clients.
- List at least five principles that form the basis of the nurse–client relationship.
- Identify the three phases of the nurse–client relationship.
- Differentiate between social communication and therapeutic verbal communication.
- Give five examples of therapeutic and non-therapeutic communication techniques.
- List at least five factors that affect oral communication.
- Describe the four forms of non-verbal communication.
- Differentiate task-related touch from affective touch.
- List at least five situations in which affective touch may be appropriate.

SECTION II: ASSESSING YOUR UNDERSTANDING

Activity A *Fill in the blanks.*

1. A(n) _____ is an association between two or more people.

2. _____ is an intuitive awareness of what a client is experiencing.

3. A(n) _____ is one who works with others to achieve a common goal.

4. A(n) _____ is one who assigns a task to someone; he or she must know what tasks are legal and appropriate for particular health care workers to perform.

5. The nurse–client relationship can be called a(n) _____ relationship.

6. The relationship between client and nurse begins with the _____ phase.

7. _____ communication is the exchange of information without using words.

8. _____ is vocal sounds that are not actually words but convey meaning.

9. _____ is as important during communication as speaking.

10. The _____ phase is a period when the relationship comes to an end.

Activity B *Consider the following figure.*

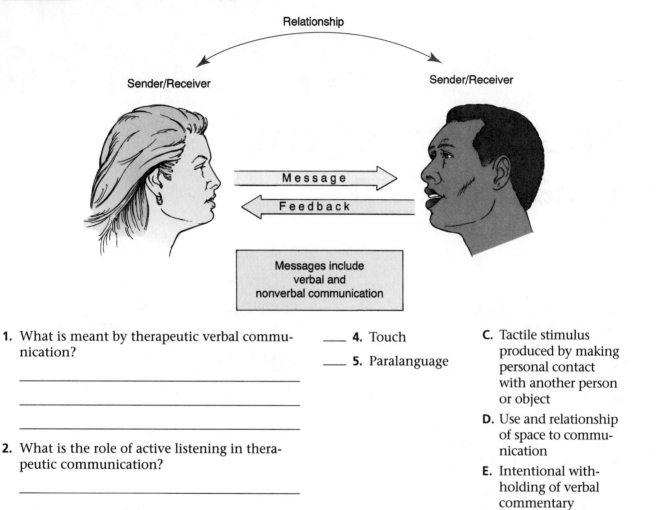

Relationship

Sender/Receiver

Sender/Receiver

Message

Feedback

Messages include
verbal and
nonverbal communication

1. What is meant by therapeutic verbal communication?

   _____

   _____

   _____

2. What is the role of active listening in therapeutic communication?

   _____

   _____

   _____

____ 4. Touch

____ 5. Paralanguage

C. Tactile stimulus produced by making personal contact with another person or object

D. Use and relationship of space to communication

E. Intentional withholding of verbal commentary

Activity C *Match the techniques of communication in column A with their description in column B.*

Column A

____ 1. Kinesics

____ 2. Silence

____ 3. Proxemics

Column B

A. Vocal sounds that are not actually words but communicate a message

B. Body language that includes non-verbal techniques such as facial expressions, posture, gestures, and body movements

Activity D *Presented here, in random order, are steps that occur during a client's stay in the hospital. Write the correct sequence in the boxes provided.*

1. Admission to the nursing unit

2. Discharge from the unit

3. Treatment and recovery

4. Diagnosis of the disease condition

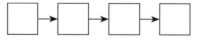

Activity E *Briefly answer the following.*

1. What are the various roles of the nurse?

   _____

   _____

   _____

2. What is meant by a therapeutic relationship?

_____

_____

_____

3. What are the phases of a nurse–client relationship?

_____

_____

_____

4. What are the factors that affect the ability to communicate by speech or in writing?

_____

_____

_____

5. What is non-verbal communication?

_____

_____

_____

Activity F *Use the clues to complete the crossword puzzle.*

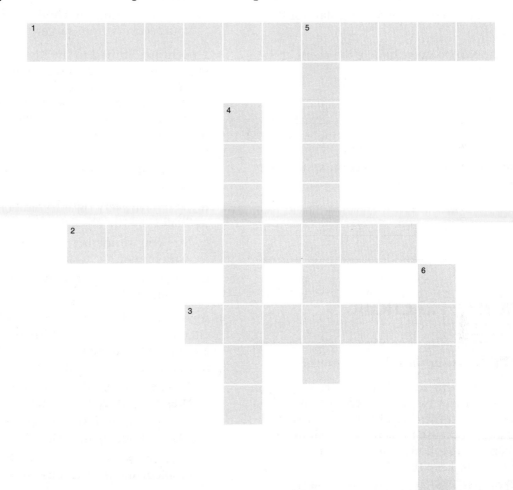

Across

1. Phase of getting acquainted
2. Set, measurable distances between people as they interact
3. Intentionally withholding verbal commentary

Down

4. Interpretation of body language, such as facial expressions and gestures
5. One who performs health-related activities that a sick person cannot perform independently
6. Type of communication using words

SECTION III: APPLYING YOUR KNOWLEDGE

Activity G *Therapeutic verbal communication refers to using words and gestures to accomplish a particular objective. It is extremely important, especially when the nurse is exploring problems with the client or encouraging expression of feelings. Answer the following questions, which involve the nurse's role when communicating with the client.*

A client is informed by the physician that his leg needs to be amputated because of a diabetic ulcer. The client is distraught and begins to cry. He is angry and blames the nursing staff for the amputation.

1. How should the nurse handle the client at this stage?

   _____

   _____

   _____

2. What should be the nurse's action to help the client deal with the loss?

   _____

   _____

   _____

SECTION IV: PRACTICING FOR NCLEX

Activity H *Answer the following questions.*

1. A nurse is caring for a client who is recovering from a cerebrovascular accident. The nurse discovers that the client has become irritable and angry because his activities are limited. Which of the following is the best nursing approach to keep the client motivated?

   a. Ignore the behavior, knowing that the client is grieving

   b. Use supportive statements to correct the client's behavior

   c. Allow frequent and longer visits by family members

   d. Tell the client that nurses know how the client feels

2. A post-operative client has been vomiting. The physician diagnoses him as having paralytic ileus and advises the insertion of a nasogastric tube. The nurse explains the purpose and steps of the procedure to the client. The client expresses that he is fed up with the treatment and cannot take it any longer. What should be the most appropriate nursing response?

   a. "If you don't have this tube inserted, you will keep on vomiting."

   b. "You have every right to refuse the treatment. Shall I call the physician?"

   c. "Get this nasogastric tube inserted and you will feel a lot better."

   d. "Are you feeling tired and frustrated with your recovery from surgery?"

3. A client is admitted to the health care facility with bowel obstruction secondary to Crohn's disease and has to undergo surgery. The client expresses his concern about whether surgery would cure his condition permanently. Which of the following is the most appropriate therapeutic statement?

   a. "Let us give this surgery a chance. You may improve."

   b. "You have every right to refuse surgery. Shall I call the physician?"

   c. "Are you wondering if this surgery will work for you?"

   d. "I have seen a similar case that was cured by surgery."

4. A new parent is trying to decide whether to circumcise her baby boy. Which is the most appropriate statement to help the parents decide about the circumcision?

   a. "Read this pamphlet and then we can talk later if you have any doubts."

   b. "The physician is the best person to give advice about circumcision."

   c. "I got my son circumcised without any problem and he is healthy now."

   d. "I would certainly recommend it, because it prevents cancer and sexually transmitted diseases."

5. A nurse in a neonatal intensive care unit is caring for a newborn diagnosed with neonatal jaundice. Which of the following statements by the nurse are most appropriate to the parents?

   a. "The baby is very sick and the next 24 hours are crucial for the baby."

   b. "The baby care unit has all the necessary equipment to take care of the baby."

   c. "Ask me any questions that you have regarding baby care."

   d. "This is common in neonates, so you should not get worried."

6. A school nurse is conducting a health education program for high school children about sexually transmitted diseases. What should be the nurse's opening statement to encourage student participation?

   a. The objective of the session is to obtain knowledge about sexually transmitted diseases

   b. Feel free to share your personal experience with the class to learn more

   c. At the end of the class, everyone should fill out a questionnaire survey form

   d. The topic is very personal, so whatever we discuss here will be kept confidential

7. A client confides to the nurse that he knows he is going to die and really wishes his family would stop hoping for a cure. He feels angry and frustrated when he sees his family trying their best. Which of the following statements is the best therapeutic response?

   a. "We should talk more about your anger toward your family."

   b. "You feel angry that your family hopes for your cure?"

   c. "It sounds as if you are being very pessimistic."

   d. "Have you shared your feelings with your family?"

8. A nurse is caring for an elderly client. The client tells the nurse that he would rather speak to the physician than talk to a mere nurse. What should be the nurse's immediate response?

   a. "I am your nurse and not your servant."

   b. "Would you prefer to speak to your physician?"

   c. "I will leave you now and call your physician."

   d. "Your physician placed you in my hands."

9. A teenage client tells the nurse that she is unhappy with herself because she is unable to do anything right. What should be the nurse's appropriate action?

   a. "You don't do anything right?"

   b. "You always do things right."

   c. "Everything will get better."

   d. "You must be holding up well."

10. A client with suicidal thoughts admits to the nurse that he does not find any reason to live and would like to end it all. Which of the following responses would help the nurse to assess the client further?

    a. "Did you have a good sleep last night?"

    b. "Tell me what you mean by that."

    c. "I am sure your family cares for you."

    d. "I know you had a stressful night."

11. A nurse is caring for a toddler who has recovered from a seizure. The mother is worried that the seizure may recur again. Which of the following is the most therapeutic statement?

    a. "Most children will never experience a second seizure."

    b. "Medicines can prevent the occurrence of seizures."

    c. "Why worry about something that you cannot control?"

    d. "Tell me more about what frightens you about seizures."

12. A client expresses to the nurse that the physician purposefully provided wrong information about his physical condition. Which of the following statements would prevent effective communication?

    a. "I am not sure to what information you are referring."

    b. "I am certain that the physician will not lie to you."

    c. "Do you want to talk to the physician again to clarify issues?"

    d. "Describe the information to which you are referring."

13. The nurse is caring for a client who is in depression and expresses that he wishes to die because he feels like a failure. What should be the best therapeutic response?

    a. "Have you been feeling like a failure for some time now?"

    b. "I see a lot of positive things in you."

    c. "It is the result of your illness that you feel this way."

    d. "You have so many purposes in life to live for."

14. A client who has been diagnosed with renal failure asks the nurse if the diagnosis means that he will die soon. What should be the nurse's immediate response?

    a. "You will do just fine."

    b. "What are you thinking about?"

    c. "You sound discouraged today."

    d. "Death is a beautiful experience."

15. A nurse is caring for a client with urticaria and pruritus. The client expresses her concern because she will be getting married within a week. She is worried about having rashes and itching. What would be the nurse's most appropriate action?

    a. "The medications will help a lot to reduce the rashes."

    b. "You are worried that this will extend into your marriage?"

    c. "It is probably just the result of pre-wedding tensions."

    d. "I hope that your husband-to-be is aware of it."

Client Teaching

SECTION I: LEARNING OBJECTIVES

■ Describe the three domains of learning.
■ Discuss three age-related categories of learners.
■ Discuss at least five characteristics unique to older adult learners.
■ Identify at least four factors that nurses assess before teaching clients.

SECTION II: ASSESSING YOUR UNDERSTANDING

Activity A *Fill in the blanks.*

1. To implement effective teaching, the nurse must determine the client's _____.

2. Teaching generally focuses on a combination of subject areas such as _____ instructions and rehabilitation programs.

3. It is essential to determine the client's level of _____ before developing a teaching plan.

4. The best teaching and learning takes place when both are _____.

5. _____ refers to the client's physical and physiologic well-being.

6. _____ is optimal when a person has a purpose for acquiring new information.

7. _____ teaching is unplanned and occurs spontaneously at the bedside.

8. Learning depends on a person's _____ and developmental level.

9. "_____ generation" refers to people born after 1981; they are also called *cyberkids*.

10. _____ illiterate people are those who possess minimal literacy skills.

Activity B *Consider the following figure.*

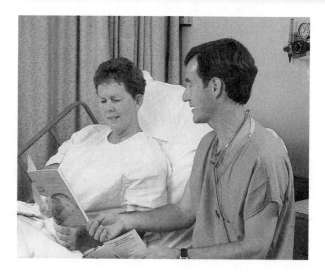

1. Identify the style of learning from the figure.

_____

_____

_____

2. What are the other styles of learning?

_____

_____

_____

Activity C *Match the learning styles in column A with their description in column B.*

Column A

____ **1.** Cognitive

____ **2.** Affective

____ **3.** Psychomotor

Column B

A. It means learning using feelings, beliefs, or values

B. It means learning by doing

C. It means learning by listening or reading facts and descriptions

Activity D *A client visits a health care facility for a session on blood sugar testing. Presented here, in random order, are steps that the nurse should perform before and during the session. Write the correct sequence of the steps in the boxes provided.*

1. Show how to take the test to evaluate the blood sugar level

2. Demonstrate the blood sugar test on a client

3. Create charts and diagrams

4. Explain why the blood sugar level increases

5. Plan how to make the session effective

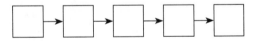

Activity E *Briefly answer the following.*

1. Explain briefly the stages of learning.

_____

_____

_____

2. What should the nurse keep in mind while implementing effective teaching to a client?

_____

_____

_____

3. What is meant by learning styles? Describe briefly the three styles of learning.

_____

_____

_____

4. Describe briefly the science involved in teaching learners of different age groups.

_____

_____

_____

5. Describe briefly the three types of age groups. What are the common learning characteristics for people born into the computer age?

_____

_____

_____

6. How do you define functionally illiterate? Give an example.

_____

_____

_____

Activity F *Use the clues to complete the crossword puzzle.*

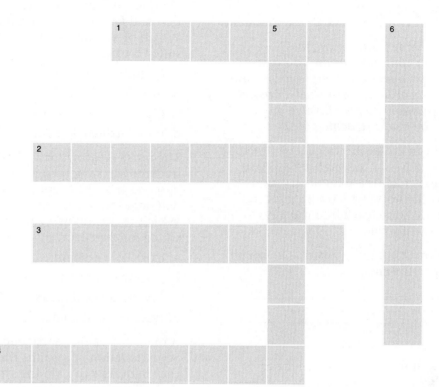

Across

1. Type of teaching that requires a plan
2. A person who cannot read and write
3. Technique of teaching children or those with cognitive ability comparable with children
4. Techniques that enhance learning among older adults

Down

5. Principles of teaching adult learners
6. Referring to the Net Generation; those born after 1981

SECTION III: APPLYING YOUR KNOWLEDGE

Activity G *Teaching is one of the most important uses of communication for nurses. Health teaching promotes the client's independent ability to meet his or her health needs. Answer the following questions, which involve the nurse's role in the health teaching of the client.*

A client brought to the health care facility with symptoms of food poisoning has been asked by the physician to get admitted for observation and treatment. The nurse who is caring for the client has been asked to teach him the ways to achieve a healthy lifestyle.

1. What question should the nurse ask to assess the learning of the client?

_____

_____

_____

2. What points should the nurse include to ensure complete health teaching before the discharge of the client?

_____

_____

_____

SECTION IV: PRACTICING FOR NCLEX

Activity H *Answer the following questions.*

1. A nurse is caring for a client with influenza and is imparting health teaching to the client. Which of the following will help the client retain the key points of the teaching?
   a. The nurse helps the client in self-administration of medications
   b. The nurse gives the client a pamphlet on how to clear nasal debris
   c. The nurse shows the client how to measure body temperature
   d. The nurse explains how to use a nebulizer mask

2. The nurse, caring for a 45-year-old client, observes that the client has very low motivation and feels that he cannot be cured. Which of the following learning styles is best suited for the client?
   a. Cognitive domain
   b. Affective domain
   c. Psychomotor domain
   d. Interpersonal domain

3. The nurse is caring for a client who has to undergo hip surgery in a week. The nurse observes that the client likes to watch videos and demonstrations, and is an avid reader. Which of the following learning styles is best suited for the client?
   a. Cognitive domain
   b. Affective domain
   c. Psychomotor domain
   d. Interpersonal domain

4. A nurse is teaching a diabetic client the self-administration of insulin. The nurse shows the client how to hold the syringe and read the calibration. This learning style is a part of which learning domain?
   a. Cognitive domain
   b. Affective domain
   c. Psychomotor domain
   d. Interpersonal domain

5. The nurse is caring for an 8-year-old client who has been admitted to the health care facility with tonsillitis. Which of the following teaching methods should the nurse use for this client?
   a. Show enthusiasm
   b. Use colorful materials
   c. Vary tone and pitch
   d. Use the client's name frequently

6. A 25-year-old client has been admitted to the health care facility for hernioplasty. Which of the following teaching methods is best suited for the client?
   a. Limit the teaching session to no longer than 15 to 20 minutes
   b. Offer praise and encouragement for accomplishments
   c. Provide the client with your total attention
   d. Assess previous learning and literacy abilities of the client

7. A 73-year-old client has been admitted to a health care facility with abdominal pains. Which of the following teaching methods is best suited for the client?
   a. Involve the client during the teaching session to impart learning
   b. Implement the teaching session when the client is most alert and comfortable
   c. Use diagrams to aid teaching during the teaching session
   d. Motivate the client to understand the importance and benefits of the session

8. The nurse is caring for a 65-year-old client with complaints of eye infection. Which of the following will help in better health teaching?
   a. Obtain pamphlets in large print
   b. Speak in a louder tone
   c. Use flash cards
   d. Select red print on white paper

9. While teaching an adult client, which of the following techniques will help the nurse to implement the health teaching better?
   a. Collaborate with the client on content
   b. Determine the client's learning style
   c. Begin with basic concepts
   d. Divide information into manageable amounts

10. A nurse involves an adult client actively in the health teaching by encouraging feedback and handling of equipment. In which of the following phases should this activity take place?
    a. Assessment
    b. Planning
    c. Implementation
    d. Evaluation

11. The nurse observes that the client's behavior consists of the following features: supporting, accepting, refusing, and defending. In which of the following learning domains do the client's learning styles fall?
    a. Cognitive domain
    b. Affective domain
    c. Psychomotor domain
    d. Interpersonal domain

12. The nurse motivates the client and promises a reward when the client can name the number of recommended servings in each category within the food pyramid. Which age category does the client likely belong to?
    a. Child
    b. Adult
    c. Older adult
    d. Net Generation

13. A nurse is caring for a client from Generation Y. Which of the following learning characteristics do clients from Generation Y share with Generation X and the Net Generation?
    a. Craving for stimulation and quick response
    b. Enthusiastic about performing repetitive tasks
    c. Preference for verbal or practical methods of participatory learning
    d. Avoidance of choosing a variety of instructional methods

14. When teaching a client the benefits of following proper toilet hygiene, the nurse observes that the client is fatigued, has low energy levels, and is not able to pay proper attention to the health teaching. Which age category does the client likely belong to?
    a. Child
    b. Adult
    c. Older adult
    d. Net Generation

15. When the nurse asks the client what she wants to accomplish at the end of the health training, which of the following is being assessed by the nurse?
    a. Preferred learning style
    b. Capacity to learn
    c. Learning readiness
    d. Learning needs

16. The nurse is caring for a 7-year-old client. Which of the following are characteristics of a pedagogic learner? Select all that apply.
    a. Lack of experience
    b. Physically mature
    c. Rote learning
    d. Responds to competition
    e. Crisis learner

17. The nurse is caring for a 73-year-old client who has been admitted to the health care facility with a slipped disc. Which of the following are characteristics of a gerogogic learner? Select all that apply.

a. Vast experience

b. Learning is self-centered

c. Needs direction and supervision

d. Responds to family encouragement

e. Long-term retention

18. The nurse is caring for a 40-year-old client who has been diagnosed with asthma. Which of the following are characteristics of an androgogic learner? Select all that apply.

a. Vast experience

b. Prefers simulation

c. Needs direction and supervision

d. Responds to family encouragement

e. Long-term retention

f. Physically mature

19. The nurse is caring for a 5-year-old client with diarrhea. Which of the following teaching styles is best suited for this client? Select all that apply.

a. Show enthusiasm

b. Use colorful materials

c. Vary tone and pitch

d. Use the client's name frequently

e. Limit the teaching session to no longer than 15 to 20 minutes

f. Offer praise and encouragement for accomplishments

g. Assess previous learning and literacy abilities

Recording and Reporting

SECTION I: LEARNING OBJECTIVES

- Identify seven uses for medical records.
- List six components generally found in any client's medical record.
- Differentiate between source-oriented records and problem-oriented records.
- Identify six methods of charting.
- Explain the purpose and applications associated with the Health Insurance Portability and Accountability Act (HIPAA).
- List four aspects of documentation required in the medical records of all clients cared for in acute settings.
- Discuss why it is important to use only approved abbreviations when charting.
- Explain how to convert traditional time to military time.
- List at least 10 guidelines that apply to charting.
- Identify four written forms used to communicate information about clients.
- List five ways that health care workers exchange client information other than by reading the medical record.

SECTION II: ASSESSING YOUR UNDERSTANDING

Activity A *Fill in the blanks.*

1. Source-oriented records generally used a(n) _____ style of charting.

2. _____ charting is most useful for nurses when a terminal is available at the point of care or at the beside.

3. _____ time is based on a 24-hour clock.

4. Charting by exception is a method in which nurses chart only _____ assessment findings.

5. The HIPAA legislation was introduced to protect the privacy of _____ records.

6. Auditors examine client medical records to determine whether the care provided meets established criteria for _____.

7. _____ charting is a modified form of SOAP charting.

8. Nurses use _____ to avoid documenting types of care that are regularly repeated.

9. When agencies can release private health information without the client's prior authorization, it is called _____ disclosures.

10. According to HIPAA rules, client information is _____ when transmitting via the Internet.

Activity B *Consider the following figure.*

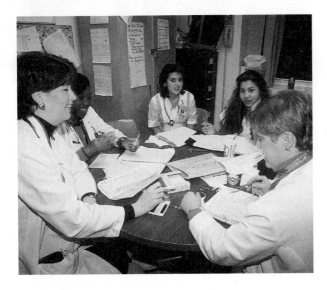

1. Identify the figure.

_____

_____

_____

2. Explain the need for this procedure.

_____

_____

_____

Activity C *Match the methods of charting in column A with their features in column B.*

Column A

_____ **1.** Narrative charting

_____ **2.** SOAP charting

_____ **3.** Computerized charting

Column B

A. Recording the client's progress under the headings of problem, intervention, and evaluation

B. Writing information about the client and client care in chronologic order

C. Documenting style more likely to be used in problem-oriented records

_____ **4.** PIE charting

_____ **5.** Charting by exception

D. Documenting abnormal assessment findings

E. Documenting the client information electronically

Activity D *Presented here, in random order, are steps taken by a nurse when exchanging information using the telephone. Write the correct sequence in the boxes provided.*

1. Identifies himself or herself by name, title, and nursing unit.

2. Obtains or states the reason for the call.

3. Repeats information to ensure it has been heard accurately.

4. Answers as promptly as possible.

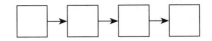

Activity E *Briefly answer the following.*

1. What are the uses of maintaining a medical record?

_____

_____

_____

2. What evidence does the Joint Commission on Accreditation of Healthcare Organizations (JCAHO) need to provide a health care facility with accreditation?

_____

_____

_____

3. How is the medical record maintained and who is responsible for maintaining the records?

_____

_____

_____

4. What care should the nurse take when documenting the medical records?

_____

_____

_____

5. What are the different methods of communicating a client's health-related details to other personnel of the agency?

_____

_____

_____

Activity F _Use the clues to complete the crossword puzzle._

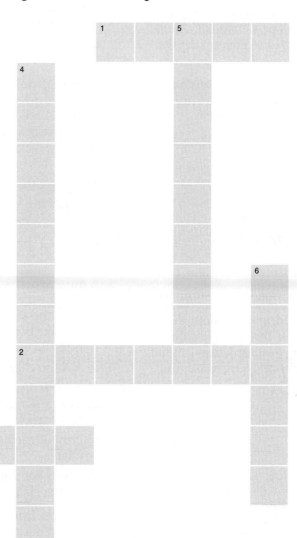

Across

1. Method of charting that believes that the word _problem_ carries negative connotations

2. A person who surveys medical records to determine whether the care provided meets established criteria for reimbursement

3. Method of recording the client's progress under the headings of problem, intervention, and evaluation

Down

4. A means of shortening the length of documentation

5. A form of documentation in which a nurse indicates with initials the performance of routine task

6. Quick reference for current information about the client and his or her care

SECTION III: APPLYING YOUR KNOWLEDGE

Activity G *Many health care facilities maintain computerized health records for their clients. Answer the following question, which involves the nurse's role in keeping client health records confidential.*

A nurse at a health care facility uses the computer to store the health records for all the clients. All nurses caring for a particular client and using the system are required to ensure that the records are confidential.

1. What care should the nurse take to ensure that these data are not available to unauthorized personnel and are not misused?

_____

_____

_____

SECTION IV: PRACTICING FOR NCLEX

Activity H *Answer the following questions.*

1. A nurse documents information about the client and client care in chronologic order in the format resembling a log or journal. What method of documentation is the nurse following in this case?
   a. SOAP charting
   b. Narrative charting
   c. PIE charting
   d. Focus charting

2. A nurse needs to access a client's data stored on a computer by a colleague. Which of the following would the nurse require to access the data from the computer?
   a. Password
   b. User name
   c. Employee identification (ID)
   d. Name

3. A nurse caring for a client documents information regarding health care in the medical record. For which of the following can the medical record be used without client's permission?
   a. Sharing information among the client's health care personnel
   b. Sharing information with personnel involved in research
   c. Sharing the client's health condition with the client's relatives
   d. Sharing the client's health condition with insurance agencies

4. A nurse caring for clients at the health care facility knows that which of the following methods can be used to obtain information on the health care provided to clients and also to serve as legal evidence during malpractice lawsuits?
   a. Calling the client's nurse for verification
   b. Checking with the other staff
   c. Checking the nursing Kardex
   d. Calling the client's physician for verification

5. A nurse who has just taken charge in the shift is caring for a client who complains of severe pain in the abdomen. What care should the nurse take before administering any medication to the client?
   a. Ask the client when he last took pain medication
   b. Check the medical record for details of medication
   c. Provide medication as requested by the client
   d. Check for the severity of pain experienced by the client

6. An officer from JCAHO is visiting the health clinic. What are the possible reasons for the officer's visit to the health clinic?
   a. To discuss the career plan with all the staff of the clinic
   b. To discuss an employee-related medical problem from JCAHO
   c. To inspect the health care agencies for the level of facilities provided
   d. To inspect the health care agencies for the evidence of quality care

7. A nurse is caring for a client with hypertension in a health care facility. The client's family observes the nurse diligently maintaining the health record and is curious to know the importance of this record for the client. Which of the following information should the nurse provide on the importance of a health record for a client?

   a. It verifies care through quality assurance programs

   b. It helps in employment and disability applications

   c. It helps in providing safe and effective care

   d. It helps in meeting standards of care set by the government

8. A nurse caring for a client is aware that the medical record of a client is an important document required by the insurance company for reimbursing the medical expenses incurred by the client. In what case can the insurance company reject the client's claim for reimbursement?

   a. Absence of health care personnel signatures

   b. Documents shared with family

   c. Documents shared with researchers

   d. Presence of abbreviated instructions

9. If a client's medical record contains separate forms on which physicians, nurses, dietitians, and physical therapists make written entries about their own specific activities related to the client's care, which method is the clinic following in organizing data?

   a. Problem-oriented records

   b. Source-oriented records

   c. PIE-charting records

   d. Focus-charting records

10. A health agency compiles and arranges all the client information according to the client's health problems. It also emphasizes goal-directed care to promote recording of pertinent information and to facilitate communication among health care professionals. Which method do you think the clinic is following in organizing data?

    a. Problem-oriented records

    b. Source-oriented records

    c. Narrative charting

    d. Computerized charting

11. A nurse records information about the client and client care under four different components—the data base, the problem list, the plan of care, and progress notes—and stores all these records in one location. Which style is the nurse using to record information in the client's record?

    a. Focus charting

    b. SOAP charting

    c. Narrative charting

    d. PIE charting

12. A nurse uses the PIE charting method for recording the information about a client. Which of the following is a feature of the PIE method?

    a. The client's listed problems are given corresponding numbers

    b. Assessments made are documented on one form

    c. The entries are in the same location in the chart

    d. The data are organized according to the client's health problems

13. A health agency has been functioning for more than 6 months and has been treating a number of clients. The next step for the health agency would be to obtain accreditation. Which of the following points should the agency keep in mind while applying for accreditation? Select all that apply.

    a. The medical records should show the nursing diagnoses or client needs

    b. The number of people working in the health agency should be more than 50

    c. The planned nursing standards of care for meeting the client's nursing care needs

    d. The latest equipment should be available to treat all kinds of health issues

    e. The client's response to interventions and outcomes of care for pain management

14. A health agency is following the computerized charting method to store data electronically. This method is useful when there is a computer terminal available at the point of care or bedside. Which of the following are advantages of computerized charting method? Select all that apply.

a. It automatically records the date and time of the documentation

b. It reduces overtime costs for uncompleted end-of-shift charting

c. The expense of purchasing a computer system is minimal

d. The abbreviations and terms are consistent with agency-approved lists

e. Electronic data require less storage space and are quickly retrievable

15. The medication order for a client states "a.c." What does "a.c." indicate?

a. Before meals

b. After meals

c. By mouth

d. Bedtime

16. A medical record states that the client has had his last medication at 1400 HR. The nurse needs to enter this detail in the computer. How should the nurse document this information in traditional time?

a. 02:00 p.m.

b. 12:00 a.m.

c. 01:40 p.m.

d. 04:00 p.m.

CHAPTER 10

Asepsis

SECTION I: LEARNING OBJECTIVES

- Describe microorganisms.
- Name eight specific types of microorganisms.
- Differentiate between non-pathogens and pathogens, resident and transient microorganisms, and aerobic and anaerobic microorganisms.
- Give two examples of the ways some microorganisms have adapted for their survival.
- Name the six components of the chain of infection.
- Cite examples of biologic defense mechanisms.
- Define nosocomial infection.
- Discuss the concept of asepsis.
- Differentiate between medical and surgical asepsis.
- Identify at least three principles of medical asepsis.
- List five examples of medical aseptic practices.
- Name at least three techniques for sterilizing equipment.
- Identify at least three principles of surgical asepsis.
- List at least three nursing activities that require application of the principles of surgical asepsis.

SECTION II: ASSESSING YOUR UNDERSTANDING

Activity A *Fill in the blanks.*

1. The most effective method for preventing infections is _____, an essential nursing activity that must be performed repeatedly when caring for clients.

2. _____, living animals or plants that are visible only with a microscope, are commonly called *germs*.

3. _____ lives abundantly and perpetually on and in the human body, which is their host.

4. Pathogens have _____, which are tiny hairs that prevent pathogens from being eliminated during urination.

5. Pathogens may cause _____ when the host is immunosuppressed from acquired immune deficiency syndrome (AIDS), cancer chemotherapy, or steroid drug therapy.

6. The three types of fungal (mycotic) infections are superficial, intermediate, and _____.

7. Helminths are classified into three major groups: nematodes, trematodes, and _____.

8. Peracetic acid is a combination of _____ acid and hydrogen peroxide.

9. Normal saline is a(n) _____ solution.

Activity B *Consider the following figure.*

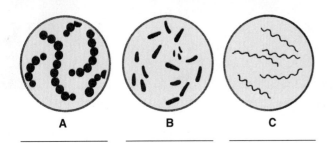

A   B   C

_____   _____   _____

1. Identify and label the figure. Give the scientific names for each.

   _____

   _____

   _____

2. What are the two types of bacteria?

   _____

   _____

   _____

3. Which type of drug is used most often to combat bacterial infections?

   _____

   _____

   _____

Activity C *Match the garments health care personnel don in column A with their functions and features in column B.*

Column A

____ 1. Gloves

____ 2. Hair and shoe covers

____ 3. Protective eyewear

Column B

A. Helps when working in the nursery, operating room, and delivery room

B. Helps reduce the spread of microorganisms onto or from the surface of clothing worn from home

C. Helps reduce transmission of pathogens present on the hair or shoes

____ 4. Clean laboratory coat

____ 5. Scrub suits or gowns

D. Helps when there is a potential transfer of microorganisms from one client or object to another client during subsequent nursing care

E. Helps when there is a possibility that body fluids will splash into the eyes

Activity D *Presented here, in random order, are the six essential components of the chain of infection. Write the correct sequence that enables the spread of disease-producing microorganisms from one location or person to another in the boxes provided.*

1. A port of entry

2. An infectious agent

3. A mode of transmission

4. A reservoir for growth and reproduction

5. An exit route from the reservoir

6. A susceptible host

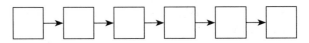

Activity E *Briefly answer the following.*

1. What are the factors that influence the development of an infection or an infectious disease in the human body?

   _____

   _____

   _____

2. What are the various types of viruses?

   _____

   _____

   _____

3. What are rickettsiae?

   _____

   _____

   _____

4. What are the classifications of protozoans?

_____

_____

_____

5. Why are mycoplasmas termed *pleomorphic?*

_____

_____

_____

6. Define and list examples of the types of biologic defense mechanisms.

_____

_____

_____

Activity F *Use the clues to complete the crossword puzzle.*

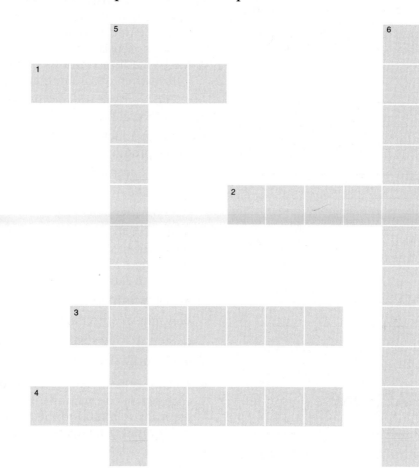

Across

1. A protein containing no nucleic acid
2. Covers to prevent droplet and airborne transmission of microorganisms
3. A practice to decrease or eliminate infectious agents, their reservoirs, and vehicles for transmission
4. A whiplike appendage needed for movement

Down

5. A microbe resembling bacteria, but it cannot survive outside another living species
6. A type of agent that inhibits the growth of but does not kill microorganisms

SECTION III: APPLYING YOUR KNOWLEDGE

Activity G *Asepsis means practices to decrease or eliminate infectious agents, their reservoirs, and vehicles for transmission. It is the major method for controlling infection. Answer the following questions, which involve the various aspects of asepsis that a nurse should follow while caring for clients.*

A nurse practices medical and surgical asepsis to accomplish care for a client suffering from an infection. There are other clients around who should be protected from the spread of infection.

1. What are the principles or measures the nurse should follow to break the chain of infection?

   _____

   _____

   _____

2. What are antimicrobial agents?

   _____

   _____

   _____

3. Which antimicrobial agents should the nurse use and why? Define the role of each type of agent.

   _____

   _____

   _____

SECTION IV: PRACTICING FOR NCLEX

Activity H *Answer the following questions.*

1. A nurse visits a client at his home. While preparing to clean her hands at the wash basin, the nurse notices a bar of soap and towel that are shared by the entire family. To prevent the spread of germs and infection, the nurse performs hand antisepsis with an alcohol-based hand rub instead of a hand wash. The nurse explains the advantages of an alcohol-based hand rub to the curious family members of the client. Which of the following is a benefit of an alcohol-based hand rub that the nurse should explain?

   a. Destroys active microorganisms but not spores

   b. Provides the fastest and greatest reduction in microbial counts on the skin

   c. Leads to irritation and drying of the skin compared with soap

   d. Controls viral replication or release from the infected cells

2. A nurse is preparing to attend an emergency case at the health clinic. Because of a lack of time, the nurse follows a faster process of hand antisepsis with an alcohol-based hand rub. What interventions should the nurse follow when decontaminating?

   a. Dip hands in the product for a minimum of 15 seconds

   b. Apply a nickel- to a quarter-size volume of the product

   c. Apply anti-infection drugs to the product

   d. Remove the product from the clean utility room

3. A nurse visits a client at the client's home; the client has a skin infection. Which of the following is the most important suggestion the nurse can give the client?

   a. Apply antiseptics

   b. Apply an antiviral lotion

   c. Stop sharing soaps, towels, and washcloths

   d. Use only sterilized instruments

4. A client is being taken to the labor room with severe contractions. The nurse has to get ready to attend to the client, who might be required to be operated. What kind of medical asepsis or cleaning technique should the nurse follow?

   a. A hand wash

   b. A hand antisepsis

   c. A surgical scrub

   d. A sterile technique

5. A nurse is supervising the performance of the housekeeping personnel in the clients' environment to check whether the principles of medical asepsis or concurrent disinfection are being carried out appropriately. What are the most important aspects the nurse should check to confirm compliance of concurrent disinfection?

   a. That the mattress and the insides of the drawers are scrubbed

   b. That the grossly soiled areas are cleaned before the less dirty ones

   c. That the floors are wet mopped and furniture is damp dusted

   d. That the contaminated equipment is boiled for 15 minutes at 212°F (100°C)

6. A nurse assisting in the operation theater is responsible for supervising the cleaning and sterilization of sharp instruments and reusable syringes. These instruments also include items that are not made of stainless steel. Which of the following methods is the most dependable for the nurse to use for physical sterilization?

   a. Using radiation

   b. Using boiling water

   c. Using free-flowing steam

   d. Using dry heat

7. A nurse is required to sterilize reusable syringes using boiling water. What is the right combination of time and temperature the nurse should use to make the sterilization process effective, given the nurse is located 100 m above sea level?

   a. Exactly 15 minutes at 112°F

   b. More than 15 minutes at 212°F

   c. Exactly 15 minutes at 100°F

   d. Less than 15 minutes at 202°F

8. The nurse in charge of the operating theater is responsible for sterilizing reusable syringes, stainless steel equipment, and heat-sensitive instruments for an operation that is due to start in less than an hour. The nurse may use chemical sterilization using gas, liquid, or physical sterilization processes. Which of the following methods should the nurse use for best results achieved as fast as possible?

   a. Gas sterilization using ethylene oxide gas

   b. Physical sterilization using steam under pressure

   c. Chemical sterilization using peracetic acid

   d. Physical sterilization using free-flowing steam

9. A nurse dons examination gloves to attend to a client admitted with a severe injury. Latex causes the nurse to suffer from skin rash, flushing, and itching. Which of the following set of gloves should the nurse don when handling the client's injury?

   a. A pair of latex gloves

   b. A pair of vinyl gloves

   c. A double pair of latex gloves

   d. A double pair of vinyl gloves

10. A nurse is handling a saline water bottle to sterilize used equipment and syringes. Which of the following interventions should the nurse follow while using the sterile solution?

   a. Hold the container below waist level while pouring

   b. Keep the cap upside down on a flat surface or hold it during pouring

   c. Pour a small amount of solution at a time to avoid contamination

   d. Touch only sterile areas within the field

11. A nurse needs to use a new scalpel for an operation. It is important that the nurse checks all the new equipment packages that have arrived in the health agency. Which of the following agency-sterilized surgical instruments should a nurse consider safe from contamination?

   a. A partially unwrapped sterile package

   b. An item sterilized a few days back

   c. A dry sterile wrapper

   d. A wet sterile wrapper

12. A nurse is attending a long-term resident client with an invasive indwelling catheter attached. Which of the following practices should the nurse follow to prevent any urinary tract infection?

   a. The tubing should always be placed higher than the bladder

   b. The tubing should never be placed higher than the bladder

   c. The tubing should never be placed at the same level as the bladder

   d. The tubing should never be placed lower than the bladder

13. A nurse is attending a 65-year-old client at the client's home. Which of the following practices should the nurse suggest that the client's family should follow to prevent the outbreak of any infection?

    a. Receive an initial dose of the pneumococcal vaccine
    b. All family members wear masks
    c. Limit personal contact with the client
    d. Provide multivitamin capsules between meals

14. A nurse is teaching an elderly female client about the ways to prevent urinary tract infections. Which of the following is the most relevant teaching?

    a. Wash and clean from the urinary area back toward the rectal area
    b. Use dry tissue to clean the urinary area
    c. Maintain dry vaginal skin
    d. Wear gloves while cleaning the urinary area

15. There is a sudden outbreak of infections at a health care facility. The nurse in charge has to start moving clients who are more susceptible to infections immediately to a safer environment. Who of the following should be moved first?

    a. Clients admitted for pathologic tests
    b. Clients with burn injuries
    c. Clients waiting for a surgery
    d. Clients who have just given birth

16. A nurse follows a set order when sterilizing all used equipment and syringes. Which of the following techniques should the nurse use to sterilize equipment? Select all that apply.

    a. Physical sterilization
    b. Chemical-dipped cloth
    c. Radiation
    d. Boiling water
    e. Dry heat

17. What points should the nurse bear in mind when sterilizing surgical equipment with peracetic acid? Select all that apply.

    a. Leads to corrosion
    b. Takes 60 minutes from start to finish

c. Sterilizes equipment quickly
d. Takes 12 minutes at 122 to 131°F
e. Takes 30 minutes from start to finish
f. Takes 30 minutes at 122 to 131°F

18. A nurse is using ethylene oxide gas to sterilize all the instruments used during a surgery. Apart from destroying the microorganisms, which of the following features should the nurse remember when working with ethylene oxide? Select all that apply.

    a. Dipped in the product for a minimum of 15 seconds
    b. Items are exposed for 3 hours at 86°F (30°C)
    c. Must be aired for a week at room temperature
    d. Must be aired for 5 days at room temperature
    e. Must be aired for 8 hours at 248°F (120°C)

19. A nurse is unwrapping a sterile package that has been delivered to the health care facility. Order the steps that the nurse should follow to unwrap the sterilized items in the most likely sequence in which they would occur.

    a. The nurse unwraps the cloth by supporting the wrapped item in one hand
    b. The nurse drops the sterile contents onto the sterile field
    c. The nurse then holds each of the four corners
    d. The nurse separates the flaps
    e. The nurse discards the cloth cover
    f. The nurse places the unwrapped item on the sterile field

20. A nurse is using the dry heat technique to sterilize sharp instruments used during a surgery. To destroy microorganisms with dry heat, the nurse needs to maintain a temperatures of 330 to 340°F for how many hours?

    a. 3 hours
    b. 2 hours
    c. Half an hour
    d. 1 hour

Admission, Discharge, Transfer, and Referrals

SECTION I: LEARNING OBJECTIVES

- List four major steps involved in the admission process.
- Identify four common psychosocial responses when clients are admitted to a health agency.
- List the steps involved in the discharge process.
- Give three examples of the use of transfers in client care.
- Explain the difference between transferring clients and referring clients.
- Describe three levels of care that nursing homes provide.
- Discuss the purpose of a minimum data set (MDS).
- Identify two contributing factors to the increased demand for home health care.

SECTION II: ASSESSING YOUR UNDERSTANDING

Activity A *Fill in the blanks.*

1. The process of entering a health care agency for nursing care and medical or surgical treatment is called _____.

2. A(n) _____ card is a plastic card delivered along with the form initiated in the admitting department to the nursing unit.

3. The envelope containing the secured valuables of the client should have the signature of the nurse, the security personnel, or the _____.

4. Termination of care from a health care agency is called _____.

5. Activities involved in discharge planning ideally begin at the time of _____.

6. Discharging a client from one unit or agency and admitting him or her to another without going home in the interim is called _____.

7. To qualify for Medicare benefits in a nursing home, a person must have been hospitalized for _____ days or more.

8. A(n) _____ care facility is a type of agency that provides health-related care and services to people who do not require 24-hour nursing.

9. A(n) _____ is the process of sending someone to another person or agency for special services.

10. A person who needs skilled nursing care intermittently will get the nursing treatment every day to once every _____ days.

Activity B *Consider the following figure.*

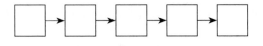

1. Identify the object in the figure.

_____

_____

_____

2. What information does this object contain?

_____

_____

_____

3. What is the use of this element?

_____

_____

_____

Activity C *Match the terms in column A with their definitions in column B.*

Column A

____ 1. Anxiety

____ 2. Against medical advice

____ 3. Transfer summary

____ 4. Extended care facility

____ 5. Basic care facility

Column B

A. Providing long-term health care

B. Leaving before the physician authorizes the discharge

C. Feeling caused by insecurity that makes the client uncomfortable

D. Providing extended custodial care

E. Briefly writing the client's current condition at the time of relocation

Activity D *Presented here, in random order, are steps occurring during the admission process. Write the correct sequence in the boxes provided.*

1. Completion of the agency's admission database

2. Documentation of the client's medical history

3. Authorization from a physician

4. Developing the initial nursing care plan

5. Collection of billing information

☐ → ☐ → ☐ → ☐ → ☐

Presented here, in random order, are steps to be followed by the nurse when helping a client undress. Write the correct sequence in the boxes provided below.

1. Remove the client's shoes

2. Cover the client with a bath blanket

3. Lift the client's head to guide garments over it

4. Release fasteners such as zippers and buttons

5. Provide privacy

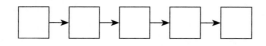

Activity E *Briefly answer the following.*

1. What is the relevance of an addressograph plate?

_____

_____

_____

2. What is an initial nursing plan?

_____

_____

_____

3. What does the medical history and physical examination generally include?

_____

_____

_____

4. What does the discharge process include?

_____

_____

_____

5. When and why does a transfer process take place?

_____

_____

_____

6. What is an extended care facility?

_____

_____

_____

Activity F *Use the clues to complete the crossword puzzle.*

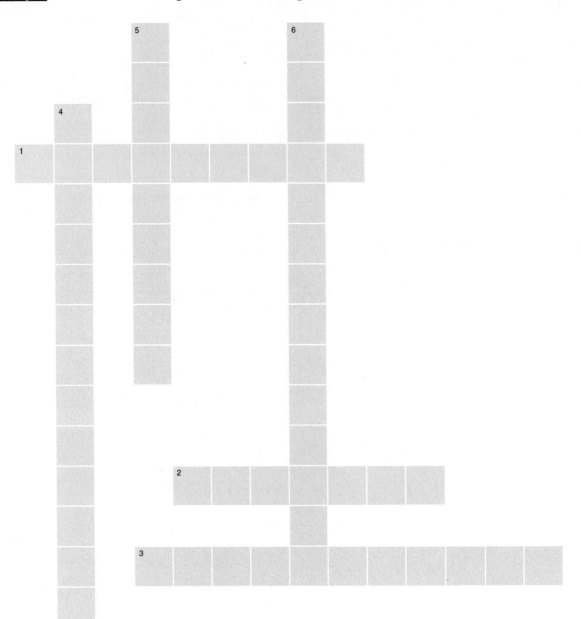

Across

1. A department where they prepare a form with the client's address, place of employment, and so forth
2. A vague uneasy feeling of discomfort or dread
3. A means of helping a person become familiar with a new environment

Down

4. Card identifying the pages within the client's medical record
5. The process of entering and staying at a health care agency for nursing care and medical or surgical treatment
6. A bracelet for the client that contains the client's name, an identification number, and a bar code for computerized scanning purposes

SECTION III: APPLYING YOUR KNOWLEDGE

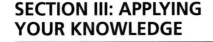 *Clients in a health care facility may be required to be transferred from one nursing unit to another within the health care facility. Answer the following questions, which involve the nurse's role in transfer of clients.*

A nurse is caring for a client who is to be shifted from the cardiac care unit to the general nursing care unit within the facility.

1. What are the nurse's responsibilities with regard to transfer of this client?

   _____

   _____

   _____

2. What does a transfer summary contain?

   _____

   _____

   _____

SECTION IV: PRACTICING FOR NCLEX

Activity H *Answer the following questions.*

1. A client who had been undergoing treatment at the health care facility has been provided with detailed instructions regarding how the medications are to be taken at home after leaving the facility. What term does the nurse use to refer to the process of sending the client home?
   a. Discharge
   b. Rule out
   c. Return
   d. Defer

2. A nurse's role includes admission and discharge procedures for clients. When preparing the discharge plan for clients, the nurse knows that which of the following clients will have special considerations and many details on their care?
   a. Clients who are 25 to 30 years old
   b. Clients with a terminal health condition
   c. Clients living with their families
   d. Clients living with relatives

3. A client wants to leave the health care facility before obtaining a discharge by the physician. The client is asked to sign a form and complete all the discharge formalities before leaving. What is the purpose of this form?
   a. To ensure that the client takes all his medications on time
   b. To ensure that the client pays all his bills before leaving
   c. To verify all the contact information of the client
   d. To release the physician and facility from future complications

4. A client who is not too happy with the type and kind of treatment being given in the health care facility decides to leave. The nurse requests him to sign a form stating that the doctor or the facility will not be responsible for any complications arising after the client is discharged. The client refuses to sign the form. What can the nurse do in this case?
   a. The nurse can note in the client's medical record that the client refused to sign the form
   b. The nurse can get the form signed by the head of the agency
   c. The nurse can sign the form herself and note that the client refused to sign it
   d. The nurse can get the form signed by the client's relative

5. A nurse has instructed the client on the medication and self-care practices to be followed after discharge from the facility. What is the next step the nurse will take to complete the discharge process?
   a. Notify the physician
   b. Notify the head of the facility
   c. Notify the business office
   d. Notify the housekeeping staff

6. A client needs to take the health care facility's transportation van after being discharged from the health agency because he is alone and not in a position to drive himself. How much time in advance does the client need to book the transportation van to use it?
   a. 2 hours in advance
   b. 6 hours in advance
   c. 12 hours in advance
   d. 24 hours in advance

7. A nurse has received orders for the transfer of a client. For which of the following reasons would a client be shifted to another agency? Select all that apply

   a. To facilitate specialized care in life-threatening conditions

   b. To provide care for the change in the client's condition

   c. To reduce the health care costs involved

   d. To provide room for another client at the facility

   e. To provide long-term care to a client after discharge

8. A client is asked to complete a form before admission to a health care agency. The form will determine the level of care the client will have while in the agency. Which of the following will the health care agency take into account to decide the level of treatment for the client? Select all that apply.

   a. Vision patterns

   b. Oral and nutritional status

   c. Financial status

   d. Mood and behavior patterns

   e. Continence patterns in the past month

9. A nurse is required to arrange for transfer of a client to another unit at the health care agency. Arrange the sequence of action required for a transfer within the agency.

   a. Speak with a nurse on the transfer unit to coordinate the transfer

   b. Transport the client and his or her belongings, medications, nursing supplies, and chart to the other unit

   c. Inform the client and family about the transfer

   d. Complete a transfer summary that briefly describes the client's current condition and reason for transfer

10. A 5-year-old child with a high fever is admitted to the health care facility. The child is scared of being in a new place with strangers and is throwing tantrums, making it difficult to care for him. How can the nurse help this child?

    a. Ask a colleague to help in feeding the child

    b. Prevent the parents from fussing over the child

    c. Provide the child with toys and books

    d. Ask a colleague to help in dressing the child

11. A client has been admitted to the health care facility for treatment of a fractured leg. He has a few personal items such as his eyeglasses. Which of the following should the nurse do for the client regarding his personal belongings?

    a. Place them on the bedside table or drawer and inform the client of this

    b. Hand them over to the client's family for safekeeping

    c. Keep them in the facility's safe along with other valuables

    d. Tell the client that the facility is not liable for client's possessions

12. Sometimes a client may need to be transferred from one unit to another unit of the health care facility. In which of the following cases would the client need to be transferred to another unit?

    a. A client who has just delivered a baby

    b. A client who is capable of going home to self-care

    c. A client who returns after leaving the facility without information

    d. A client who might leave the facility against medical advice

CHAPTER 12

Vital Signs

SECTION I: LEARNING OBJECTIVES

- List four physiologic components measured during the assessment of vital signs.
- Differentiate between shell and core body temperature.
- Identify the two scales used to measure temperature.
- List four temperature assessment sites and indicate the site considered the closest to core temperature.
- Name four types of clinical thermometers.
- Discuss the difference between fever and hyperthermia.
- Name the four phases of a fever.
- List at least four signs or symptoms that accompany a fever.
- Give two reasons for using an infrared tympanic thermometer when body temperature is subnormal.
- List at least four signs and symptoms that accompany subnormal body temperature.
- Identify three characteristics noted when assessing a client's pulse.
- Name the most commonly used site for pulse assessment and three other assessment techniques that may be used.
- Name and explain at least four terms used to describe abnormal breathing characteristics.
- Discuss the physiologic data that can be inferred from a blood pressure assessment.
- Explain the difference between systolic and diastolic blood pressure.
- Name three pieces of equipment for assessing blood pressure.
- Describe the five phases of Korotkoff sounds.
- Identify three alternative techniques for assessing blood pressure.

SECTION II: ASSESSING YOUR UNDERSTANDING

Activity A *Fill in the blanks.*

1. _____ is a term used to describe a warmer-than-normal set point.

2. A(n) _____ scale is used in the United States to measure and report body temperature.

3. _____ is a structure within the brain that helps control various metabolic activities and acts as the center for temperature regulation.

4. _____ stiffens body hairs and gives the appearance of what commonly is described as "goose flesh."

5. _____ rhythms are physiologic changes, such as fluctuations in body temperature and other vital signs, that happen during 24-hour cycles.

6. _____ affect metabolic rate by triggering hormonal changes through the sympathetic and parasympathetic pathways of the autonomic nervous system.

7. The _____, or the underarm, is an alternative site for assessing body temperature.

8. A(n) _____ thermometer uses a temperature-sensitive probe covered with a disposable sheath and attached by a coiled wire to a display unit.

9. A(n) _____ ultrasound device is an electronic instrument that detects the movement of blood through peripheral blood vessels and converts the movement to a sound.

10. _____ sounds result from the vibrations of blood within the arterial wall or changes in blood flow.

Activity B *Consider the following figures.*

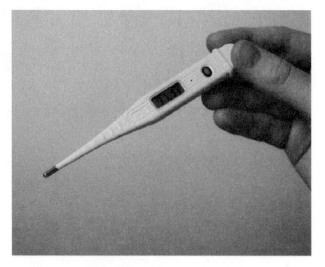

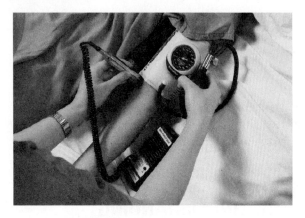

1. Identify the equipment.

_____

_____

_____

2. Explain the use of this equipment.

_____

_____

_____

3. Identify the equipment.

_____

_____

_____

4. Describe the equipment.

_____

_____

_____

Activity C *Match the terms related to measuring vital signs in column A with their descriptions in column B.*

Column A	Column B
____ **1.** Tachypnea	**A.** Cooling of the ear when it comes in contact with the probe of the thermometer
____ **2.** Bradycardia	
____ **3.** Drawdown effect	**B.** Use of calories for sustaining body functions
____ **4.** Metabolic rate	**C.** Rapid respiratory rate
____ **5.** Hypotension	**D.** Blood pressure measurements are below the normal systolic values for the person's age
	E. Pulse rate is less than 60 bpm

Activity D *Presented here, in random order, are four distinct phases through which fever progresses. Write the correct route in the boxes provided.*

1. Invasion phase
2. Defervescence phase
3. Prodromal phase
4. Stationary phase

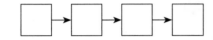

Activity E *Briefly answer the following.*

1. What is systolic pressure?

   _____

   _____

   _____

2. What should the nurse do if the client's temperature is not normal?

   _____

   _____

3. What are objective assessment data?

   _____

   _____

   _____

4. What causes an increase in body temperature during ovulation?

   _____

   _____

   _____

5. How does emotion affect body temperature?

   _____

   _____

6. When is a paper chemical thermometer used?

   _____

   _____

   _____

Activity F *Use the clues to complete the crossword puzzle.*

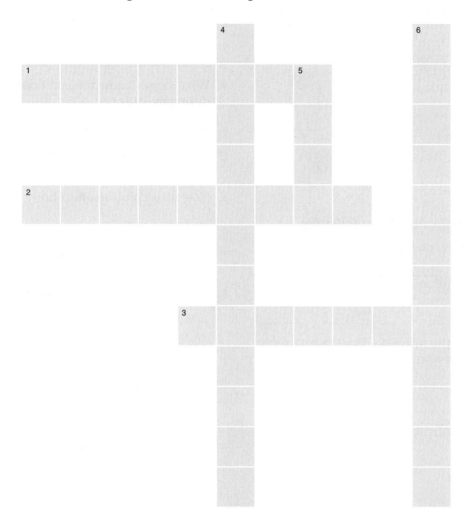

Across

1. An infrared thermometer is also referred to as this

2. Slower-than-normal respiratory rate at rest

3. A condition in which body temperature is elevated

Down

4. Drugs that reduce fever

5. Warmth in deeper sites within the body like the brain and the heart

6. Excessively high core temperature

SECTION III: APPLYING YOUR KNOWLEDGE

Activity G *Shell temperature in normal, healthy adults generally ranges from 96.6 to 99.3°F (35.8–37.4°C). On the other hand, the core body temperature ranges from 97.5 to 100.4°F (36.4–37.3°C). The nurse measures the temperature of the client routinely. Answer the following questions, which involve the nurse's role in the physical assessment of clients.*

A nurse is caring for a client with a high fever. The nurse notices that the client is shivering and his body is hot. The nurse has been instructed by the physician to record the client's body temperature regularly.

1. How should the nurse ensure that the temperature measured reflects the core body temperature?

   _____

   _____

   _____

2. How should the nurse document the different assessment sites in the client's medical record?

   _____

   _____

   _____

SECTION IV: PRACTICING FOR NCLEX

Activity H *Answer the following questions.*

1. A nurse is regularly assessing the temperature of a client with hyperthermia. At what temperature would the chances for survival of a client be diminished?
   a. Body temperatures exceeding 120°F or falling below 95°F
   b. Body temperatures exceeding 105°F or falling below 84°F
   c. Body temperatures exceeding 110°F or falling below 84°F
   d. Body temperatures exceeding 115°F or falling below 95°F

2. When assessing the temperature of a client after the afternoon meal, the nurse notes an increase in the temperature of the client from the last assessment. Which of following conditions could have led to the increase in the client's temperature in this case?
   a. The client was sleeping during the day
   b. The amount and type of food eaten
   c. The client has a rapid respiratory rate
   d. The medication used by the client

3. A nurse is caring for an asthmatic client at the health agency. The nurse notes an increase in the client's temperature after the client has taken his medication. Which of the following medications could have possibly led to an increase in the client's body temperature?
   a. Aspirin
   b. Ibuprofen
   c. Ephedrine
   d. Acetaminophen

4. A nurse needs to measure the body temperature of an infant client. From which of the following sites should the nurse measure the infant's temperature?
   a. Oral
   b. Rectal
   c. Ear
   d. Axillary

5. The nurse is caring for a 26-year-old female client. When measuring her temperature, the nurse notes an increase in the body temperature of the client, even though she shows no symptoms of fever. Which of the following conditions could have led to an increase in temperature in the client?
   a. Lack of perspiration
   b. Depression
   c. Ovulation
   d. Use of aspirin

6. When assessing the client, the nurse notes that the slightest bit of pressure obliterates the client's pulse. How should the nurse record the client's pulse?
   a. Bounding
   b. Thready
   c. Strong
   d. Normal

7. A nurse is caring for a client who was in a mountaineering accident. The nurse should assess the client for which of the following symptoms of hypothermia?
   a. Increased metabolic demand
   b. Irregular breathing rhythm
   c. Above-normal pulse rates
   d. Impaired muscle coordination

8. A nurse is caring for an adult client with a body temperature of 103.4°F. Which of the following would be an appropriate nursing intervention for this client?
   a. Provide fluids
   b. Provide aspirin
   c. Provide physical cooling
   d. Suggest rest

9. A nurse is caring for a client with dyspnea. The nurse should note which of the following conditions could bring about dyspnea in a client?
   a. The amount and type of activity
   b. The eating habits of the client
   c. The regularity with which it occurs
   d. The hours the client sleeps

10. A nurse uses the aneroid manometer to check the blood pressure of the client. What should the nurse check for before measuring the blood pressure?
    a. The needle on the gauge must be positioned at zero
    b. The gauge reading must be same as the client's body temperature
    c. The gauge is connected to an electric outlet
    d. The inflatable bladder must be of the correct size

11. A nurse is caring for a client whose blood flow in the arteries is very low. The nurse has to use the Doppler ultrasound device to detect the movement of blood through peripheral blood vessels. Order the steps in the most likely sequence in which they would occur when the nurse uses the Doppler device to assess the client's pulse rate.
    a. Move the probe at an angle over the skin
    b. Count the pulsating sound

c. Document the assessment site rate
d. Apply conductive gel over the arterial site
e. Note the "D" for Doppler device

12. A nurse needs to measure the blood pressure of a client from a site other than the brachial artery. In which of the following cases would the nurse need to use an assessment site other than the brachial artery? Select all that apply.
    a. When the client's arms are missing
    b. When both breasts have been removed
    c. When a client has had vascular surgery
    d. When the client has hypothermia
    e. When the client is moderately hypothermic

13. A nurse is caring for a client with low blood pressure. Identify the situations in which a client could have low blood pressure? Select all that apply.
    a. Increasing age
    b. Sleeping at night
    c. Lying down posture
    d. Client is a female
    e. Exercise and activity

14. A nurse needs to assess the blood pressure of an elderly client. Order the steps in the most likely sequence in which they would have occurred when measuring the blood pressure of the client.
    a. Have the client assume a sitting position
    b. Assist the client to stand and check the pressure
    c. Assess the blood pressure with the client in the supine position
    d. Deflate and leave the blood pressure cuff in place
    e. Check the client's blood pressure

15. A nurse is measuring the Korotkoff's sound in a client. Which of the following phase of Korotkoff's sounds appears to be muffled, less distinct, and softer with a blowing quality?
    a. Phase I
    b. Phase II
    c. Phase III
    d. Phase IV

CHAPTER 13

Physical Assessment

SECTION I: LEARNING OBJECTIVES

■ List four purposes of a physical assessment.
■ Name four assessment techniques.
■ List at least five items needed when performing a basic physical assessment.
■ Discuss at least three criteria for an appropriate assessment environment.
■ Identify at least five assessments that can be obtained during the initial survey of clients.
■ State two reasons for draping clients.
■ Differentiate between a head-to-toe and a body systems approach to physical assessment.
■ List six ways in which the body may be divided for organizing data collection.
■ Identify two self-examinations that nurses should teach their adult clients.

SECTION II: ASSESSING YOUR UNDERSTANDING

Activity A *Fill in the blanks.*

1. The overall goal of a physical assessment is to gather _____ data about a client.

2. A(n) _____ is an instrument used to examine structures in the eye.

3. A(n) _____ is a professional trained to test hearing with standardized instruments.

4. _____ is an exaggerated natural lumbar curve of the spine.

5. _____ is excessive fluid within tissue, and signifies abnormal fluid distribution.

6. The yellowish brown, waxy secretion produced by glands within the ear is called _____.

7. A(n) _____ chart is a visual assessment tool with small print.

8. The _____ test is an assessment technique for comparing air versus bone conduction of sound.

9. _____ is a combination of the elastic quality of the skin and the pressure exerted on it by fluid within.

10. A(n) _____ test is an assessment technique for determining equality or disparity of bone-conducted sound.

Activity B *Consider the following figures.*

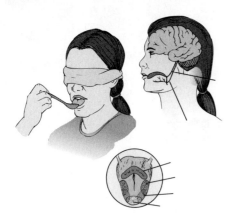

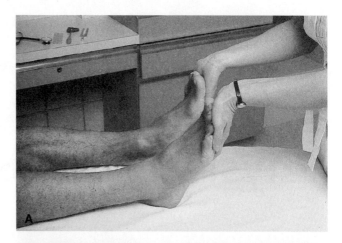

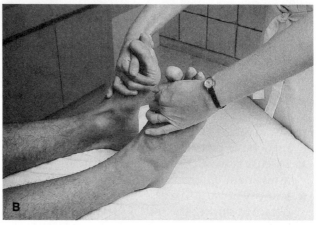

1. Identify and label the figure.

_____

_____

_____

2. How is a taste assessment done?

_____

_____

_____

3. How does the nurse ensure valid results when assessing taste in a client?

_____

_____

_____

4. Identify the figure.

_____

_____

_____

5. How is this procedure performed?

_____

_____

_____

Activity C *Match the terms related to assessment of the eye in column A with their descriptions in column B.*

Column A

___ **1.** Visual acuity

___ **2.** Normal vision

___ **3.** Consensual response

___ **4.** Visual field examination

___ **5.** Accommodation of pupils

Column B

A. Ability to read printed letters at a distance of 20 feet without prescription lenses

B. Assessment of peripheral vision and continuity in the visual field

C. Ability to see both far and near

D. Ability to constrict when looking at a near object and dilate when looking at an object in the distance

E. Brisk, equal, and simultaneous constriction of both pupils when one eye, and then the other, is stimulated with light

Activity D *Presented here, in random order, are steps occurring during the assessment of pupillary response. Write the correct sequence in the boxes provided.*

1. Repeat the assessment by directly stimulating the opposite eye.

2. Ask the client to look at a finger or object approximately 4 inches from his or her face.

3. Bring a narrow beam of light from a penlight, from the temple toward the eye.

4. Tell the client to look from the near object to another that is more distant.

5. Dim the lights in the examination area and instruct the client to stare straight ahead.

6. Observe the pupil of the stimulated eye as well as the unstimulated pupil.

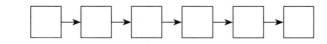

Activity E *Briefly answer the following.*

1. What is the purpose of a physical assessment?

_____

_____

_____

2. What are the basic requirements of an examination room for assessing clients?

_____

_____

_____

3. Why is it important to document the client's weight and height during an initial assessment?

_____

_____

_____

4. How should the nurse assess a client's hair?

_____

_____

_____

5. Why is it important for the nurse to document any unusual characteristics of the nails or surrounding tissues?

_____

_____

_____

6. What equipment would the nurse need for a basic physical assessment?

_____

_____

_____

Activity F *Use the clues to complete the crossword puzzle.*

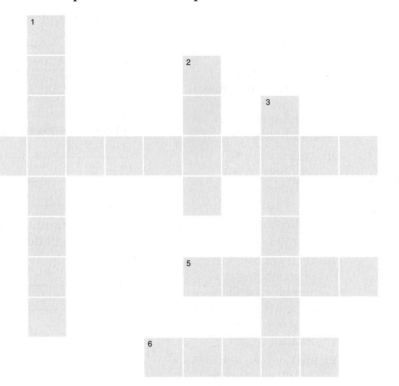

Across

4. A torn, jagged wound
5. A break in the skin
6. An open, craterlike area in the skin

Down

1. An area that has been rubbed away by friction
2. A mark left by the healing of a wound or lesion
3. A crack in the skin, especially in or near mucous membranes

SECTION III: APPLYING YOUR KNOWLEDGE

Activity G *The first step in the nursing process is assessment. The overall goal of physical assessment is to gather objective data about a client. Answer the following questions, which involve the nurse's role in the physical assessment of clients.*

A nurse is caring for a client with an abdomen that appears unusually enlarged. The nurse is assessing the bowel as part of the physical assessment.

1. In what order should the nurse use the assessment techniques?

_____

_____

_____

2. How should the nurse measure the abdominal girth of the client?

A nurse is caring for a middle-age client at the health care facility. During the physical assessment, the nurse asks the client to perform a regular testicular self-examination. The client is not aware of the method of self-examination.

3. What should the nurse tell the client with regard to the procedure for testicular self-examination?

_____

_____

_____

SECTION IV: PRACTICING FOR NCLEX

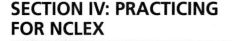 **Answer the following questions.**

1. A nurse, when conducting a physical assessment for a client, observes several lesions on the skin that are elevated, with irregular borders and no free fluid. The client informs the nurse that these lesions erupted after having shellfish. How should the nurse document this observation?

   a. Macules

   b. Papules

   c. Wheals

   d. Vesicles

2. A nurse is assessing the skin turgor of a client during a regular physical assessment. Which of the following areas is the best site to test for skin turgor?

   a. The area over the chest

   b. The area at the back of the hand

   c. The area on the forearm

   d. The area on the lower leg

3. When listening to the lung sounds of a client, the nurse hears adventitious sounds that are intermittent, high-pitched, popping sounds during inspiration. How should the nurse document these adventitious sounds?

   a. Rubs

   b. Wheezes

   c. Gurgles

   d. Crackles

4. A nurse is caring for a client at the health care facility. What should the nurse do if adventitious sounds are heard when assessing the lung sounds of the client?

   a. Assist the client to a supine position

   b. Assess the appearance of raised sputum

   c. Move the diaphragm from the base of the lung to the top

   d. Listen for one complete inspiration or expiration

5. The nurse is examining a client with complaints of pain in the abdomen. The nurse applies pressure in the abdominal region with the fingertips and the palm of the hand to check for tenderness or unusual vibrations. What kind of physical assessment technique is the nurse using to examine this client?

   a. Inspection

   b. Percussion

   c. Palpation

   d. Auscultation

6. A nurse at the health care facility is examining a client during a routine checkup. What care should the nurse do when obtaining the client's weight?

   a. Check to see that the scale is calibrated at zero

   b. Ask the client to remove his or her shoes and provide the client with light slippers

   c. Move the heavier weight across the calibrations

   d. Position the lighter weight in a calibrated groove of the scale arm

7. When performing a physical assessment for a client, a nurse should also assess the mental status of the client. In which of the following cases should the nurse perform an in-depth objective assessment? Select all that apply.

   a. Clients with head injury

   b. Clients with psychiatric diagnoses

   c. Clients with impaired visual acuity

   d. Clients who are being treated with nonsteroidal anti-inflammatory drugs (NSAIDs)

   e. Clients who took an overdose of drugs

8. A nurse is caring for a child with complaints of pain in the right ear. Which of the following steps should the nurse perform when examining the child's ear?

   a. Place the vibrating tuning fork behind the head to assess hearing

   b. Pull the ear down and back to straighten the ear canal

   c. Move the external ear to determine any tenderness

   d. Position the client in front of a diffused lamp for examination

9. During a routine physical examination, the nurse inspects the skin of the client. The nurse observes purple patches of skin on the legs of the client. How should the nurse document this finding?

a. Pallor

b. Erythema

c. Cyanosis

d. Ecchymosis

10. During a visit to the health care facility, a client in her mid 30s asks the nurse for information about breast self-examination (BSE). Which of the following should the nurse tell the client?

a. Perform self-examination once every 2 months

b. Place the hand alongside the side to be examined

c. Squeeze the nipple gently to determine whether there is any discharge

d. Perform the entire examination while lying down

11. During a routine physical assessment of a pregnant client, the nurse observes edema on the client's feet. How should the nurse document the edema, if a 4-mm pit is observed with a fairly normal contour?

a. 1+ pitting edema

b. 2+ pitting edema

c. 3+ pitting edema

d. 4+ pitting edema

12. A nurse is assessing the sensory skin perception of a client. What should the nurse do to test the client's ability to identify fine touch?

a. Place the stem of a vibrating tuning fork against the wrist

b. Touch the client with pointed and curved ends of a safety pin

c. Stroke the skin at various areas with a cotton ball

d. Touch the skin at various areas with warm and cold containers

13. A nurse is caring for a client with complaints of abdominal pain. The nurse auscultates the abdomen and feels for palpable masses. How should the nurse document the shape and consistency of an abdominal mass that resembles an egg and feels firm to the touch?

a. Round and nodular

b. Ovoid and nodular

c. Ovoid and hard

d. Round and hard

14. A nurse is assessing a client who has been having irregular bowel movements. The client also complains of heaviness and uneasiness in the abdomen. What should the nurse do when assessing the abdomen for bowel sounds?

a. Warm the diaphragm of the stethoscope before the procedure

b. Listen for 1 minute in each quadrant

c. Listen for bowel sounds in one upper and one lower quadrant

d. Explain the procedure to the client during the assessment

15. A nurse is assessing the heart sounds of a 35-year-old client with a possible heart condition. Which of the following is a normal heart sound?

a. The "lub" sound louder at the mitral area

b. The "lub-dub-dub" sounds

c. The "lub-lub-dub" sounds

d. The soft "dub" sound over the aortic area

CHAPTER 14

Special Examinations and Tests

SECTION I: LEARNING OBJECTIVES

- Differentiate between an examination and a test.
- List 10 general nursing responsibilities related to assisting with special examinations and tests.
- Name five positions commonly used during tests or examinations.
- Explain what is involved during a pelvic examination and a Pap test.
- List six commonly performed categories of tests or examinations.
- Identify four word endings and their meanings that provide clues regarding how tests or examinations are performed.
- Explain the following procedures: sigmoidoscopy, paracentesis, lumbar puncture, throat culture, and measurement of capillary blood glucose.
- Discuss at least three factors to consider when performing examinations and tests on older adults.

SECTION II: ASSESSING YOUR UNDERSTANDING

Activity A *Fill in the blanks.*

1. A consent form contains three elements: capacity, comprehension, and _____.

2. The _____ position is a reclining position with the feet in metal supports called *stirrups.*

3. _____ are samples of tissue or body fluids that are collected during an examination or test.

4. During an X-ray, the actual film image is technically called a(n) _____.

5. During a radionuclide examination, the nurse should ask clients about their allergy history because _____ is used commonly during this examination.

6. _____ is a form of radiography that displays an image in real time.

7. Visual examination of internal structures using optical scopes is known as _____.

8. Endoscopic examinations that produce discomfort or anxiety are performed under a light, short-acting form of _____, sometimes referred to as *conscious sedation.*

9. Barium retention can lead to _____, and bowel obstruction.

10. Ultrasonography is also known as _____.

Activity B *Consider the following figures.*

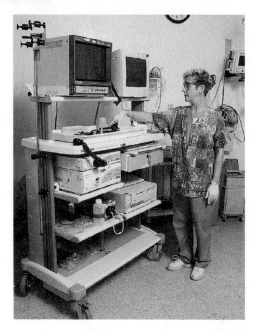

4. What is the use of the objects in the figure?

_____

_____

_____

Activity C *Match the examination in column A with their descriptions in column B.*

Column A

_____ **1.** Computed tomography

_____ **2.** Radionuclides

_____ **3.** Magnetic resonance imaging

_____ **4.** Echogram

_____ **5.** Cold spot

Column B

A. Elements with molecular structures that are altered to produce radiation

B. Technique for producing an image by using atoms subjected to a strong electromagnetic field

C. Area with little radionuclide concentration

D. Form of roentgenography that shows planes of tissues

E. Can be viewed in real time on a monitor and recorded for future analysis

1. Identify the figure.

_____

_____

2. What care should the nurse perform before the examination?

_____

_____

_____

Activity D *Presented here, in random order, are steps to collect specimens during an examination or test. Write the correct sequence in the boxes provided.*

1. Label the specimen container with the correct information.

2. Collect the specimen in an appropriate container.

3. Ensure that the specimen does not decompose before it can be examined.

4. Deliver the specimen to the laboratory as soon as possible.

5. Attach the proper laboratory request form.

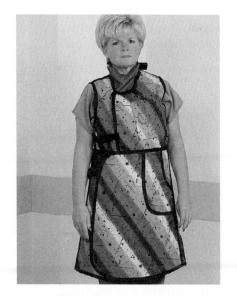

3. Identify the figure.

_____

_____

□ → □ → □ → □ → □

Activity E *Briefly answer the following.*

1. What are diagnostic examinations?

_____

_____

_____

2. What is a culture?

_____

_____

_____

3. What is a contrast medium?

_____

_____

_____

4. How is a lumbar puncture performed?

_____

_____

_____

5. What other information, in addition to a written account of the examination, should a nurse report?

_____

_____

_____

6. What care should a nurse take when attending to a client?

_____

_____

_____

Activity F *Use the clues to complete the crossword puzzle.*

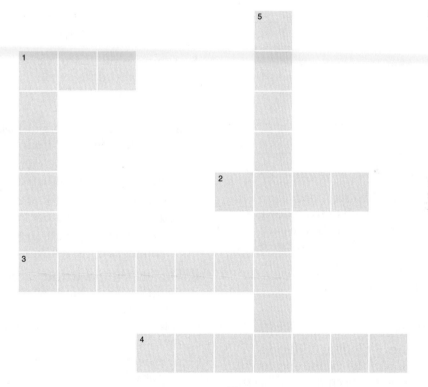

Across

1. A test during which screening of cervical cells is done
2. Position in which the client lies on the left side with the chest leaning forward
3. Incubation of microorganisms
4. Area where the radionuclide is intensely concentrated

Down

1. Type of examination that involves the physical inspection of the vagina and cervix with palpation of the uterus and ovaries
5. Samples of tissue or body fluids

SECTION III: APPLYING YOUR KNOWLEDGE

Activity G *Nursing responsibilities for a client examination include gathering information from the client before an examination and providing instructions for the client to follow after the examination. Answer the following questions, which involve the nurse's responsibilities while helping a client undergo radionuclide imaging.*

A middle-age female client needs to undergo radionuclide imaging as a part of her diagnosis.

1. What questions should the nurse ask the client before the examination?

   _____

   _____

   _____

2. What instructions should the nurse provide the client after the examination?

   _____

   _____

   _____

SECTION IV: PRACTICING FOR NCLEX

Activity H *Answer the following questions.*

1. A client visits the health care agency for a scheduled checkup. Which of the following positions should the nurse assist the client to get into to examine the client's prostate gland?

   a. Dorsal recumbent position

   b. Lithotomy position

   c. Genupectoral position

   d. Sims' position

2. A physician advises a client to undergo a physical inspection of the vagina and cervix for which the nurse has been directed to collect a specimen of cervical secretions. Which of the following tests is the client supposed to undergo?

   a. Pap smear

   b. Radiography

   c. Fluoroscopy

   d. Endoscopy

3. A client is scheduled to undergo a procedure in which an endoscope is inserted into the upper airway or upper gastrointestinal tract. For how many hours before the procedure should the nurse withhold food and fluids?

   a. At least 1 hour

   b. At least 2 hours

   c. At least 4 hours

   d. At least 6 hours

4. A client with frequent complaints of pain in the lower abdomen has been ordered to undergo an endoscopy. The client is administered conscious sedation during the procedure. Which of the following is an effect of conscious sedation?

   a. The client may not recall having had the test

   b. The client's breathing will be affected

   c. The client will be under heavy sedation

   d. The client may have a sore throat

5. A nurse is preparing a client for an endoscopic procedure of the lower intestine. What should the nurse do before this procedure?

   a. Confirm that the client has not had any food for the past 2 hours

   b. Confirm that bowel preparation using enemas has been completed

   c. Confirm that the client drank six to eight glasses of water before the examination

   d. Confirm that the client has good swallow, cough, and gag reflexes

6. In addition to a written account of the client's examination, what other primary information should the nurse record to share with the other nursing team members?

   a. Where and how the specimen was transported

   b. The client's reactions during and immediately after the procedure

   c. Where the test was performed and who performed it

   d. Type and quantity of the specimen obtained from the client

7. The nurse is assisting a client who is to undergo a paracentesis procedure. Why should the nurse encourage the client to empty the bladder just before the procedure?
   a. To prevent any accidental puncture
   b. To pool the fluids in the lower area of the abdomen
   c. To displace the intestines posteriorly
   d. To prevent contaminating the physician's sterile gloves

8. A client has been ordered an examination of the anal region. Which of the following positions should the nurse ask the client to maintain during the examination?
   a. Dorsal recumbent position
   b. Sims' position
   c. Genupectoral position
   d. Modified standing position

9. For which procedure is the nurse preparing the client if the nurse requests the client to remove all metal items (such as religious medals or clothing that contains metal objects) before the examination?
   a. Radiography
   b. Endoscopy
   c. Paracentesis
   d. Electrocardiography (ECG or EKG)

10. During the pelvic examination of a client, the nurse folds back the drape just before the examination begins. Which of the following is a possible reason for the action of the nurse?
    a. To maintain the client's modesty and privacy
    b. To reduce anxiety
    c. To expose the genitalia, minimizing exposure
    d. To illuminate the area, facilitating examination

11. A client has to undergo an examination of the energy emitted by the brain for which the client needs to be awake after midnight before the examination. What type of examination does the client have to undergo?
    a. Electroencephalography (EEG)
    b. ECG

c. Electromyography (EMG)
d. Electrodes

12. A nurse is caring for a client with respiratory disorder resulting from a collection of fluid in the lungs. For which of the following procedures would the nurse be required to assist the client?
    a. Lumbar puncture
    b. Pelvic examination
    c. Throat culture
    d. Paracentesis

13. A pregnant client visits the health agency for her scheduled checkup. Which of the following positions should the nurse assist the client to get into so that the physician can perform a gynecologic examination?
    a. Dorsal recumbent position
    b. Lithotomy position
    c. Sims' position
    d. Knee–chest position

14. A client with complaints of irritation and itching in her vaginal area visits the health agency. Which of the following tests should the client undergo to determine the cause for her condition?
    a. Blood test
    b. Ultrasound
    c. Papanicolaou test
    d. Microorganisms analysis

15. A nurse teaches a diabetic client to measure her own glucose level daily. Which of the following should the nurse tell the client is the best time to determine her blood glucose level?
    a. 30 minutes before eating and before bedtime
    b. 30 minutes after eating and before bedtime
    c. 30 minutes before eating and after waking up
    d. 30 minutes after eating and after waking up

16. A client has been ordered to have a laboratory test. Which of the following should the nurse ensure when preparing the client for a laboratory procedure? Select all that apply.

    a. The nurse should schedule the procedures before the client consumes the herbal medicine

    b. The nurse should know the client's previous results of the test as a baseline for comparison

    c. The nurse should inform the client when to stop consuming the prescribed medication

    d. The nurse must assess the blood pressure of older clients before the procedure

    e. The nurse should provide older adults with additional clothing to keep them warm

17. A frail and elderly client has to undergo a gastrointestinal examination and an examination to check blood sugar levels, which requires the client to fast for some time. The client is diabetic and also has a breathing problem. What special care should the nurse take when scheduling the tests for this client? Select all that apply.

    a. Suggest the client fasts for 8 hours before the tests

    b. Eliminate long periods of fasting during the tests

    c. Suggest the client fast for 12 hours before the tests

    d. Offer food and fluid after the tests

    e. Provide a bedside commode if necessary

18. What care should the nurse take when sending a stool sample, collected from a client, to the laboratory for testing? Select all that apply.

    a. Label the specimen container with the correct information

    b. Send it to the laboratory at the earliest possible moment before it decomposes

    c. Keep changing the container so that it does not decompose

    d. Store the specimen in a refrigerator

    e. Attach the proper laboratory request form

19. A nurse is caring for a client who visits the health agency for a prostate gland examination as a part of his annual checkup. Order the tasks in the most likely sequence in which the nurse would have performed them while caring for the client.

    a. The nurse helps the client to a position of comfort

    b. The nurse directs the client to dress in their own clothing

    c. The nurse provides instructions for follow-up care

    d. The checks the client's vital signs to verify that his condition is stable

    e. The nurse escorts the client to the discharge area

    f. The nurse cleans any substances from the client that caused soiling

20. A physician needs to examine an arthritic client with complaints of pain in the vagina. The nurse helps the client to get in to the Sims' position for the examination. Which of the following positions should the nurse help the client to assume? Select all that apply.

    a. The client lies on her left side with her chest leaning forward

    b. The client's right knee is bent toward her head

    c. The client rests on her knees and chest supported by a pillow

    d. The client's head is supported on a small pillow, to one side

    e. The client's left arm is extended behind the body

CHAPTER 15

Nutrition

SECTION I: LEARNING OBJECTIVES

- Define nutrition and malnutrition.
- List six components of basic nutrition.
- List at least five factors that influence nutritional needs.
- Discuss the purpose and components of a food pyramid.
- Describe three facts available on nutritional labels.
- Explain protein complementation.
- Identify four objective assessments for determining a person's nutritional status.
- Discuss the purpose of a diet history.
- List five common problems that can be identified from a nutritional assessment.
- Plan nursing interventions for resolving problems caused or affected by nutrition.
- List seven common hospital diets.
- Discuss four nursing responsibilities for meeting clients' nutritional needs.
- Identify three facts the nurse must know about a client's diet.
- Describe and demonstrate techniques for feeding clients.
- Explain how to meet the nutritional needs of clients with visual impairment or dementia.
- Discuss at least three unique aspects of nutrition that apply to older adults.

SECTION II: ASSESSING YOUR UNDERSTANDING

Activity A *Fill in the blanks.*

1. _____ is a condition resulting from lack of proper nutrients in the diet.

2. The energy, or heat equivalent, of food is measured in _____.

3. _____ is the amount of heat that raises the temperature of 1 kg water to 1°C.

4. Cholesterol absorbs fatty acids and binds them to molecules of protein referred to as _____.

5. Carbohydrates contain _____, an indigestible fiber in the stems, skins, and leaves of fruits and vegetables.

6. _____ help to regulate many of the body's chemical processes such as blood clotting and conduction of nerve impulses.

7. _____ amino acids, which are protein components, cannot be synthesized by the body.

8. _____ fats are obtained from plant sources such as corn, safflower, olives, peanuts, and soybeans.

9. _____ is a condition associated with Alzheimer's disease and refers to the deterioration of previous intellectual capacity.

10. _____ is gas formed in the intestine and released from the rectum when eructation does not occur.

Activity B *Consider the following figure.*

Nutrition Facts

Nutrition Facts
Serving Size 1/2 of package (21g)
Servings Per Container 2

Amount Per Serving	
Calories 70	Calories from Fat 20
	% Daily Value*
Total Fat 2.5g	4%
Saturated Fat 1.5g	6%
Cholesterol Less than 5mg	1%
Sodium 940mg	39%
Total Carbohydrate 12g	4%
Dietary Fiber 1g	6%
Sugars 4g	
Protein 2g	
Vitamin A 0% •	Vitamin C 0%
Calcium 6% •	Iron 2%

* Percent Daily Values are based on 2,000
calorie diet. Your daily values may be higher
or lower depending on your calorie needs:

	Calories:	2,000	2,500
Total Fat	Less than	65g	80g
Sat Fat	Less than	20g	25g
Cholesterol	Less than	300mg	300mg
Sodium	Less than	2,400mg	2,400mg
Total carbohydrate		300g	375g
Dietary Fiber		25g	30g

Calories per gram:
Fat 9 • Carbohydrate 4 • Protein 4

1. Identify the figure.

_____

2. What does the figure display?

_____

_____

_____

3. What are daily values (DVs)?

_____

_____

_____

Activity C *Match the food nutrients in column A with their descriptions and functions in column B.*

Column A

_____ **1.** Vitamins

Column B

A. Non-caloric substances in food that help regulate many of the body's cellular functions

_____ **2.** Minerals

_____ **3.** Cholesterol

_____ **4.** Fats

_____ **5.** Carbohydrates

B. Chemical substances necessary in minute amounts for normal growth, maintenance of health, and functioning of the body

C. Chief component of most diets, and the body's primary source for quick energy

D. Absorbs fatty acids and binds them to molecules of protein referred to as *lipoproteins*

E. Concentrated energy source supplying more than twice the calories per gram than proteins

Activity D *Presented here, in random order, are steps followed for measuring midarm circumference. Write the correct sequence in the boxes provided.*

1. Find the midpoint of the upper arm between the shoulder and elbow.

2. Record the circumference in centimeters.

3. Mark the midarm location.

4. Use the non-dominant arm.

5. Position the arm loosely at the client's side.

6. Encircle the arm with a tape measure at the marked position.

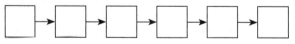

Activity E *Briefly answer the following.*

1. What are the parameters for nutritional needs?

_____

_____

_____

2. How do water-soluble vitamins differ from fat-soluble vitamins?

_____

_____

_____

_____

3. What factors influence an individual's eating habits?

_____

_____

_____

4. What should the nurse check for during the physical assessment of a client?

_____

_____

_____

5. What measures should the nurse take when feeding a visually impaired client?

_____

_____

_____

6. What are the various factors that reduce appetite and nutritional intake in older adults?

_____

_____

_____

Activity F _Use the clues to complete the crossword puzzle._

Across

1. Excessive leanness

Down

2. General wasting away of body tissue
3. Difficulty chewing and swallowing food
4. Usually precedes vomiting
5. Loss of appetite
6. A person who relies exclusively on plant sources for protein

SECTION III: APPLYING YOUR KNOWLEDGE

Activity G *Nurses use various assessment techniques and equipment to perform physical assessment. The environment must facilitate accurate data collection and be conducive to the client's privacy and comfort. Answer the following questions, which involve the nurse's role in feeding, assessment, and planning for the client.*

A nurse is caring for a client with dysphagia who has undergone a surgery for a cataract in his left eye.

1. What care should the nurse take when feeding this client?

_____

_____

_____

SECTION IV: PRACTICING FOR NCLEX

Activity H *Answer the following questions.*

1. During the assessment of a client's diet a nurse notes that the client's diet lacks enough sources of complete protein. Which of the following sources of food should the nurse recommend for ensuring complete proteins in the client's diet?
   a. Poultry
   b. Beans
   c. Nuts
   d. Grains

2. A nurse is physically assessing a client with malnutrition who belongs to an affluent family in the United States. Which of the following could be a probable reason for the client's malnutrition, taking into consideration that the client belongs to an affluent family?
   a. Eating disorders
   b. Religious beliefs
   c. History of malnutrition
   d. Emotional disorders

3. A nurse is caring for a client diagnosed with deficiency of water-soluble vitamins. Which of the following vitamins should the nurse recommend as a supplement?
   a. Vitamin A
   b. Vitamin C
   c. Vitamin D
   d. Vitamin E

4. A nurse is assessing the body-mass index of four clients diagnosed with risk of weight-related problems. Which of these clients can be categorized as obese?
   a. Client A, who has a body-mass index of 30.2 kg/m^2
   b. Client B, who has a body-mass index of 28.6 kg/m^2
   c. Client C, who has a body-mass index of 29 kg/m^2
   d. Client D, who has a body-mass index of 29.5 kg/m^2

5. A nurse is caring for a client who has been diagnosed with a blood clot in his lower left leg. Which of the following should the nurse recommend to regulate the blood-clotting processes in the client's body?
   a. Proteins
   b. Fats
   c. Carbohydrates
   d. Minerals

6. When assessing the client's dietary intake, the nurse notes that the client's daily diet exceeds 2,000 calories. Which of the following should the nurse recommend changing in the client's diet?
   a. Unsaturated fats
   b. Vitamins
   c. Cholesterol
   d. Minerals

7. A nurse is analyzing the eating habits of a female client who works in a high-profile law firm in the city. The nurse notes that the client does not include any meat or dairy products in her diet. Which factor could be influencing the client's eating habits?
   a. Access to food markets
   b. Vegetarianism
   c. Veganism
   d. Pregnancy

8. A nurse is assessing the diet of a vegan client. What is the nurse's observation about the nutrients that seems to be lacking in a vegan diet?
   a. Fats
   b. Vitamin C
   c. Protein
   d. Minerals

9. A nurse is recording the objective data of a vegetarian client. What should the nurse measure to obtain anthropometric data of the client?
   a. Height
   b. Biceps skin thickness
   c. Chest width
   d. Wrist diameter

10. A nurse is recording the dietary history of a client to obtain facts about her eating habits. Which of the following will the nurse note in the dietary history of the client?
    a. The timing of meals
    b. The protein intake
    c. The amount of cholesterol level
    d. The intake of unsaturated fats

11. A nurse is conducting a physical assessment of a client who has been admitted to the health care facility. What are the factors the nurse should check during the physical assessment?
    a. Height
    b. Diet
    c. Skin
    d. Weight

12. The nurse is caring for a visually impaired client at the health care facility. What should the nurse do when feeding a visually impaired client?
    a. Request a full liquid diet or a mechanically soft diet
    b. Provide small, frequent meals if eating efforts tire the client
    c. Determine whether the client has swallowed the food before offering another mouthful
    d. Arrange to have finger food prepared for the client

13. After completing the physical assessment of a client, the nurse notices a gag reflex in the client. Which of the following does it indicate?
    a. Dysphagia
    b. Nausea
    c. Eructation
    d. Xerostomia

14. Which of the following observations during the physical assessment of a client are indications of obesity in the client?
    a. A body-mass index of 15 or more and a triceps skinfold measurement of more than 15 mm
    b. A body-mass index of 25 or more and a triceps skinfold measurement less than 15 mm
    c. A body-mass index of 30 or more and a triceps skinfold measurement more than 15 mm
    d. A body-mass index of 35 or more and a triceps skinfold measurement more than 15 mm

15. A nurse is caring for a client with a body-mass index of 37. How can the nurse help the client to lose weight safely?
    a. Reducing the diet by 200 calories per day
    b. Reducing the diet by 1,200 calories per day
    c. Reducing the diet by 1,500 calories per day
    d. Reducing the diet by 800 calories per day

16. A nurse is assisting a client with dementia. How can the nurse ensure that the client eats the food that has been served to him? Select all that apply.
    a. Communicate visually and spatially that the client should eat the food
    b. Inform the client about the kind of food you are offering with each mouthful
    c. Ensure that the client is able to see another person eating in the vicinity
    d. Be firm with the client and insist that the client eats the food
    e. Provide small, frequent meals if efforts to eat and swallow tire the client

17. A nurse is assessing the diet of a client diagnosed with a fat-soluble vitamin deficiency. Which vitamin supplements should the nurse prescribe to cover this deficiency? Select all that apply.

   a. Vitamin A

   b. Vitamin B

   c. Vitamin C

   d. Vitamin D

   e. Vitamin E

   f. Vitamin K

18. During the physical assessment of a client, the nurse notes that the client appears exhausted and devoid of energy. The medical records indicate that the client's diet lacks carbohydrates. What can the nurse change in the diet to cover the lack of carbohydrates? Select all that apply.

   a. Increase quantity of cereals

   b. Increase quantity of grains

   c. Increase quantity of egg

   d. Increase quantity of yolk

   e. Increase quantity of meat

19. A nurse is caring for an older client with complaints of dental pains. What measures can the nurse take to remedy the oral problems that interfere with nutritional intake? Select all that apply

   a. Get dental care every 6 months

   b. Practice good dental hygiene daily

   c. Encourage drinking non-caffeinated beverages

   d. Encourage over-the-counter, herbal therapies

   e. Increase caloric intake in the diet

20. During the physical assessment of a client, the nurse records the weight of the client as 185 lbs and the height as 5 feet 4 inches. What is the body-mass index of the client?

   a. 26.3

   b. 28.2

   c. 27.4

   d. 29.0

CHAPTER 16

Fluid and Chemical Balance

SECTION I: LEARNING OBJECTIVES

- Name four components of body fluid.
- List five physiologic transport mechanisms for distributing fluid and its constituents.
- Name 10 assessments that provide data about a client's fluid status.
- Describe three methods for maintaining or restoring fluid volume.
- Describe four methods for reducing fluid volume.
- List six reasons for administering intravenous fluids.
- Differentiate between crystalloid and colloid solutions, and give examples of each.
- Explain the terms *isotonic, hypotonic,* and *hypertonic* when used in reference to intravenous solutions.
- List four factors that affect the choice of tubing used to administer intravenous solutions.
- Name three techniques for infusing intravenous solutions.
- Discuss at least five criteria for selecting a vein when administering intravenous fluid.
- List seven complications associated with intravenous fluid administration.
- Discuss two purposes for inserting an intermittent venous access device.
- Identify three differences between administering blood and crystalloid solutions.
- Name at least five types of transfusion reactions.
- Explain the concept of parenteral nutrition.

SECTION II: ASSESSING YOUR UNDERSTANDING

Activity A *Fill in the blanks.*

1. _____ is the escape of intravenous fluid into the tissue.

2. Fluid that represents the greatest proportion of water in the body is present inside the cells and is called _____ fluid.

3. Fluid present outside the cells is called _____ fluid.

4. Fluid in the tissue space between and around the cells is called _____ fluid.

5. _____ are neurologic infectious microorganisms that cause various brain disorders.

6. _____ are substances that carry either a positive or negative electrical charge.

7. A fluid deficit in both extracellular and intracellular compartments causes _____.

8. _____ tubing is necessary for administering solutions packaged in rigid glass containers.

9. _____ devices are used to access the venous system by piercing a vein with a needle.

10. _____ or the inflammation of a vein is a complication associated with the infusion of intravenous solutions.

Activity B *Consider the following figure.*

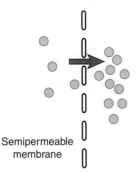

Semipermeable
membrane

1. Identify the type of distribution mechanism.

_____

_____

_____

2. How does this method help regulate the distribution of water in the body?

_____

_____

_____

3. How do colloids affect this distribution mechanism?

_____

_____

_____

Activity C *Match the terms related to fluids and chemical balance in column A with their description in column B.*

Column A

_____ **1.** Filtration

_____ **2.** Hydrostatic pressure

_____ **3.** Passive diffusion

Column B

A. Physiologic process in which dissolved substances move from an area of higher concentration to an area of lower concentration

B. Identical balance of cations with anions

C. Process in which dissolved substances require the assistance of a carrier molecule to pass from one side of a semipermeable membrane to the other

_____ **4.** Electro-chemical neutrality

_____ **5.** Facilitated diffusion

D. Regulates the movement of water and substances from a compartment where the pressure is higher to one where pressure is lower

E. Pressure exerted against a membrane

Activity D *Presented here, in random order, are mechanisms that maintain a match between fluid intake and output. Write the correct sequence in the boxes provided.*

1. Stimulates the person to drink.

2. Kidneys excrete water to maintain proper balance.

3. The brain triggers the sensation of thirst.

4. Fluid volume expands.

5. Body fluid becomes concentrated.

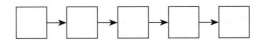

Activity E *Briefly answer the following.*

1. What is body fluid made of? What are the sources of body water?

_____

_____

_____

2. What is donated blood tested for?

_____

_____

_____

3. What is the importance of electrolytes?

_____

_____

_____

4. Who are universal donors and recipients? Which are the blood groups that come under this category?

_____

_____

_____

5. What is the importance and role of non-electrolytes?

_____

_____

_____

6. What are the differences between donor blood and blood recipient?

_____

_____

_____

Activity F *Use the clues to complete the crossword puzzle.*

Across

1. Are also known as white blood cells
2. The carrier substance for glucose

Down

3. An organ that excretes water to maintain or restore proper balance
4. Example of a substance distributed by facilitated diffusion
5. Also known as thrombocytes
6. Blood and blood products are examples of this type of solution

SECTION III: APPLYING YOUR KNOWLEDGE

Activity G *Fluid deficit occurs when there is a low volume in the extracellular fluid compartments. Fluid deficit leads to dehydration, which can be mild, moderate, and severe. Answer the following questions, which involve the nurse's role in the physical assessment of clients.*

A client is admitted to the health agency with complaints of dizziness and weakness. The client complains that he lacks the energy to perform his daily activities. The physician, on examining him, directs the nurse to put him on glucose drips.

1. What are the other symptoms that the nurse should observe in this client?

   _____

   _____

   _____

2. What nursing intervention should the nurse perform to ensure that the client's condition improves?

   _____

   _____

   _____

SECTION IV: PRACTICING FOR NCLEX

Activity H *Answer the following questions.*

1. A client with severe leg injury from an accident has been brought to the health agency. The client has lost a lot of blood and needs a transfusion. The client's blood group is A, Rh negative. Which of the following blood groups could be considered for this client (apart from A, Rh negative)?

   a. A, Rh positive

   b. O, Rh negative

   c. AB, Rh negative

   d. B, Rh positive

2. A nurse is caring for several clients at the health care facility. Which of the following clients would require fluid volume assessment?

   a. Client with tonsillitis

   b. Client with diarrhea

   c. Client with viral infection

   d. Client with jaundice

3. A client has been admitted to the health agency with complaints of loose bowel movements and vomiting that has persisted for more than a week. The client has become weak and exhausted. The nurse should note which of the following as the possible cause for the client's condition?

   a. Hypervolemia

   b. Edema

   c. Hypovolemia

   d. Hypoalbuminemia

4. During the initial assessment of a client who has been admitted to the health agency as a result of dehydration, the nurse notes a 4% loss of body weight for the client. How should the nurse document the client's level of dehydration?

   a. Moderate dehydration

   b. Severe dehydration

   c. Total dehydration

   d. Mild dehydration

5. A nurse is caring for an elderly client with a cardiovascular disorder. What should the nurse do to avoid the fluid and electrolyte imbalances that may result from the administration of diuretic medication to an elderly client?

   a. Encourage non-caffeinated beverages

   b. Encourage consumption of more food

   c. Offer caffeinated beverages every 3 hours

   d. Avoid intake of salt in food

6. A client who has been diagnosed with hypovolemic shock is being treated with plasma expanders to increase blood volume and raise his blood pressure. Which of the following products would the nurse use to get the desired outcome in this case?

   a. Dextran 40

   b. Perfluorocarbons

   c. Microencapsulated hemoglobin

   d. Hemosol

7. A client is diagnosed with body fluid in excess of 3 L. The physician directs the nurse to reduce the client's fluid intake and to administer medication that would promote urine elimination in the client. How should the nurse note the client's condition in his medical record?

   a. Edema

   b. Hypervolemia

   c. Hypovolemia

   d. Hypoalbuminemia

8. The nursing care plan indicates that a client is to be weighed regularly. Which of the following points should the nurse consider when weighing the client?

   a. Should be weighed wearing light clothes daily

   b. Should be weighed at the same time of day daily

   c. Should be weighed on a different scale to avoid discrepancy

   d. Should be weighed thrice a week at the same time

9. A client with symptoms of edema has been brought to the health agency for treatment. As part of the nursing intervention, which of the following should the nurse ensure during the care of the client?

   a. Increasing the infusing volume

   b. Increasing fluid intake

   c. Restricting salt intake

   d. Reducing sugar intake

10. A client is being treated for swelling in his tissues and fluid accumulation in the body cavity at the health agency. Per the direction of the physician, the nurse administers albumin by intravenous infusion. Which of the following nursing interventions should the nurse perform when administering the intravenous solution to the client?

    a. Infuse fluids at smaller volumes at rapid rates

    b. Monitor the client for signs of circulatory overload

    c. Infuse fluids at smaller volumes at slower rates

    d. Monitor the client for signs of dehydration

11. A client has been diagnosed with albumin deficiency in the blood. The physician directs the nurse to administer albumin by intravenous infusion to the client. Which of the following problems could arise as a result of the deficit of albumin in the client's body?

    a. Heart disease

    b. Dehydration

    c. Peritoneum infection

    d. Liver disease

12. When administering lipid emulsions to a malnourished client, the nurse observes a certain adverse reaction in the client resulting from the administration of the medication. Which of the following symptoms would the nurse observe with regard to the client's adverse reaction to the medication?

    a. Cyanosis

    b. Cardiac arrest

    c. Gall bladder enlargement

    d. Anemia

13. A physician directs the nurse to administer isotonic solution to a client who is dehydrated. Under what condition is an isotonic solution administered to the client?

    a. The client's fluid losses exceed fluid intake

    b. The client is not able to eat or drink for a short period

    c. The client's cerebral edema has to be reduced

    d. The client is not able to urinate properly

14. A client is being treated for hypovolemic shock at the health agency. The nurse knows that which of the following is used to treat hypovolemic shock?

    a. Oxygent

    b. Fluorosol DA

    c. Hespan

    d. Hemosol

15. A client is being administered an intravenous solution. The physician orders the nurse to monitor the client for any signs of complications. Which of the following are complications associated with the administration of intravenous solutions? Select all that apply.

    a. Edema

    b. Phlebitis

    c. Hypervolemia

    d. Dehydration

    e. Thrombus formation

16. A client at the health agency is receiving a blood transfusion. What nursing intervention should the nurse perform during the transfusion? Select all that apply.

    a. Release the blood from the blood bank 5 hours prior to transfusion

    b. Stay with the client for the first 15 minutes of the transfusion

    c. Squeeze and turn the container before starting the transfusion

    d. Avoid frequent assessment of the client during the transfusion

17. After weighing a client who uses a diaper, the nurse subtracts the weight of a similar dry item to record the total fluid output of the client on a daily basis. The nurse, when recording the output in milliliters, should record that 0.47 kg fluid is equal to _____ mL?

    a. 487

    b. 100

    c. 475

    d. 337

18. A nurse needs to provide a client 1 tablespoon glucose in 1 ounce water. The nurse knows that the solution prepared is _____ mL glucose with 30 mL water.

    a. 15

    b. 20

    c. 10

    d. 25

19. A nurse has been directed by the physician to give 1 ounce glucose to a client who is on an intravenous fluid intake. The nurse would need to give _____ mL glucose to the client.

    a. 10

    b. 30

    c. 20

    d. 15

Hygiene

SECTION I: LEARNING OBJECTIVES

- Define hygiene.
- Name five hygiene practices that most people perform regularly.
- Give two reasons why a partial bath is more appropriate than a daily bath for older adults.
- List at least three advantages of towel or bag baths.
- Name two situations in which shaving with a safety razor is contraindicated.
- Name three items recommended for oral hygiene.
- Identify two methods to prevent the chief hazard when providing oral hygiene to an unconscious client.
- Describe two techniques for preventing damage to dentures during cleaning.
- Describe two methods for removing hair tangles.
- Name two types of clients for whom nail care is provided with extreme caution.
- Name four visual and hearing devices.
- List two alternatives for clients who cannot insert or care for their own contact lenses.
- Discuss four reasons for sound disturbances experienced by people who wear hearing aids.
- Describe an infrared listening device.

SECTION II: ASSESSING YOUR UNDERSTANDING

ACTIVITY A *Fill in the blanks.*

1. _____ protects the layers and structures within the lower portions of the skin.

2. _____ is a slimy substance that keeps the membranes soft and moist.

3. As the jaw grows, the _____ teeth are replaced by permanent teeth.

4. The combination of sugar, plaque, and bacteria may eventually erode the tooth enamel and cause _____.

5. A contact lens is a small plastic disk placed directly on the _____ of the eye.

6. Oral hygiene consists of those practices used to clean the _____.

7. A podiatrist undergoes special training in caring for the _____.

8. Older adults are more susceptible to impacted _____, a common cause of hearing loss.

9. A(n) _____ is a person who prescribes corrective lenses.

10. The _____ layer separates the skin from skeletal muscles.

Activity B *Consider the following figures.*

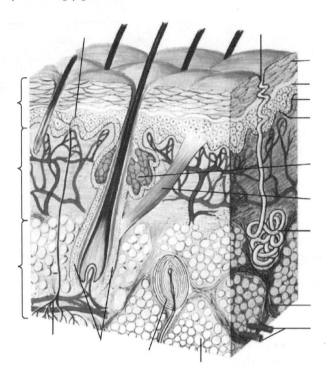

1. Identify and label the figure.

   _____

   _____

   _____

2. What are the functions of the various layers in the figure?

   _____

   _____

   _____

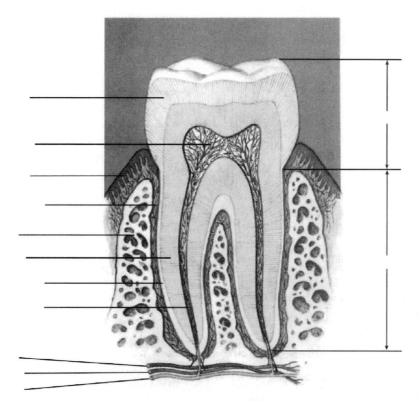

3. Identify and label the figure.

_____

_____

_____

4. List three common problems associated with this part of the body.

_____

_____

_____

Activity C *Match the terms related to hygiene in column A with their functions in column B.*

Column A

_____ **1.** Contact lenses

_____ **2.** Bathing

_____ **3.** Flossing

_____ **4.** Skin

_____ **5.** Shaving

Column B

A. Regulates body temperature

B. Reduces the potential of getting infected

C. Removes unwanted body hair

D. Placed directly on the cornea

E. Removes plaque

Activity D *Presented here, in random order, are steps that a nurse takes when providing nail care for clients. Write the correct sequence in the boxes provided.*

1. Push cuticles downward with a soft towel.

2. Soak the hands or feet in warm water.

3. Use a hand-held electric rotary file to reduce the length of long fingernails or toenails.

4. Clean under the nails with a wooden orange stick.

5. Check with the client's physician before cutting fingernails or toenails.

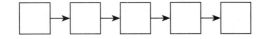

Activity E *Briefly answer the following.*

1. How should the nurse provide oral care for an unconscious client?

_____

_____

_____

2. What is a partial bath?

_____

_____

_____

3. What are the four important functions of the skin?

_____

_____

_____

4. What care should the nurse take when grooming a client's hair?

_____

_____

_____

5. What care should the nurse take when caring for the client's eyeglasses?

_____

_____

_____

Activity F *Use the clues to complete the crossword puzzle.*

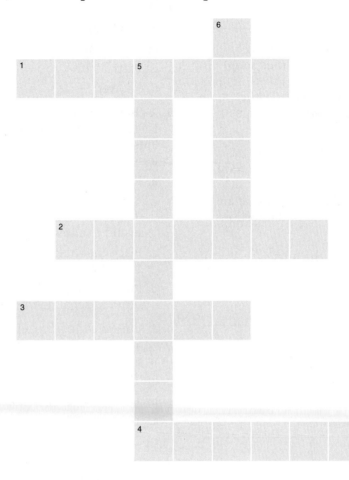

Across

1. Thin edge of skin at the base of the nail
2. Those practices that promote health through personal cleanliness
3. True skin
4. Hardened plaque

Down

5. A collective structure that covers the surface of the body
6. A substance composed of mucin and other gritty substances in saliva

SECTION III: APPLYING YOUR KNOWLEDGE

Activity G *Bathing is a hygienic practice during which a cleaning agent (such as soap) is used to remove sweat, oil, dirt, and microorganisms from the skin. Answer the following questions, which involve the nurse's role in assisting clients with bathing.*

A nurse is caring for an elderly client who has undergone rectal surgery. The client is averse to bathing daily. The nurse needs to ensure that body areas subject to greatest soiling or that are sources of body odor are cleaned and infections do not occur.

1. What kind of bath should the nurse suggest to the client?

   _____

   _____

   _____

2. What care should the nurse take when providing perineal care to the client?

   _____

   _____

   _____

SECTION IV: PRACTICING FOR NCLEX

Activity H *Answer the following questions.*

1. A nurse is caring for a client with an artificial eye. The nurse is assisting her to clean the eye. How will the nurse remove the artificial eye for cleaning?

   a. Depress the lower eyelid to remove the artificial eye

   b. Place an ophthalmic suction cup on the eye

   c. Extend the eyelid to remove the artificial eye

   d. Irrigate the eye socket

2. A nurse is caring for a 71-year-old client with acute arthritis. When caring for the client's personal hygiene, what kind of bath should the nurse consider for this client?

   a. Bed bath

   b. Towel bath

   c. Partial bath

   d. Shower

3. A client is new to wearing soft contact lenses. He is nervous and needs help to remove the lenses. How should the nurse remove the lenses?

   a. Remove the lens from the cornea to the sclera by sliding it into position

   b. Remove the lens by depressing the lower eyelid to allow the lens to slide free

   c. Place the thumb on the upper lid and use the other finger to remove the lens

   d. Press the upper lid and ask the client to blink to separate the lens

4. A nurse is caring for a client with high fever. To which temperature should the nurse heat the water to provide a towel bath for this client?

   a. 45 to 50°F

   b. 100 to 104°F

   c. 105 to 110°F

   d. 55 to 60°F

5. A nurse is caring for a young employed woman with a hearing impairment. The young woman is required to wear a hearing aid to compensate for her hearing impairment. The woman needs to travel and meet several people as part of her work. What kind of hearing aid should for the nurse suggest for this client?

   a. Behind-the-ear devices

   b. Infrared listening devices

   c. Body aid devices

   d. Canal Aids

6. A nurse is caring for an elderly client with reduced mobility. The nurse has to clean the eyeglasses of this client. She has cleaned them by running tepid water over both sides of the glass. Which of the following should she use to dry the glass?

   a. Woolen cloth

   b. Soft handkerchief

   c. Paper tissues

   d. Dryer

7. A nurse is caring for a client who has been diagnosed with cancer. The client is undergoing chemotherapy. What precaution should the nurse take when grooming his hair?

    a. Use a wide-tooth comb

    b. Ask the client to keep his hair short

    c. Brush his hair from the crown

    d. Provide a turban or cap

8. A nurse is caring for a client who is in coma. What care should the nurse take with regard to the client's oral hygiene?

    a. The nurse should use waxed floss

    b. The nurse should use sterile solution

    c. The nurse should use liquid oral hygiene

    d. The nurse should use oral swabs

9. A nurse is caring for an elderly client with limited mobility resulting from arthritis. The client has had a surgery for cataracts. How should the nurse assist the client to take care of her dentures?

    a. Clean the dentures with hot water and antiseptic solution

    b. Store the dentures in a bowl of warm water

    c. Use cotton swabs to clean the dentures

    d. Use a clean facecloth to free the dentures from the mouth

10. An elderly client needs assistance in bathing. The client refuses to have a partial bath and insists on a shower. How should the nurse help the client?

    a. Provide non-skid mat on floor

    b. Give him a towel bath

    c. Give him a bag bath

    d. Insist on a partial bath

11. A nurse is caring for a diabetic client with thick and discolored nails. How should the nurse help this client with regard to nail care?

    a. Clean the nails with warm water

    b. File and trim the client's nails

    c. Clean under the nails with a clean towel

    d. Request the services of a podiatrist

12. A nurse is caring for a female client with impaired skin on the feet. What should the nurse suggest to this client with regard to care of the skin?

    a. Instruct the client to wear leather slippers

    b. Instruct the client to wear flip-flops

    c. Instruct the client to wear sturdy slippers

    d. Instruct the client to wear heeled shoes

13. A nurse is assessing an elderly client with brown, flat patches on the face, hands, and forearms. How should the nurse document this finding?

    a. Seborrheic keratoses

    b. Senile lentigines

    c. Scleroderma

    d. Acne

14. A nurse is caring for an elderly client who is frail. The nurse provides a bed bath to the client to provide hygiene. What care should the nurse take when providing a bed bath for the client? Select all that apply.

    a. Use different towels to clean different parts of the body

    b. Clean from the feet and move upward

    c. Air-dry the skin for 2 to 3 seconds

    d. Fold the soiled areas of the towel to the outside

    e. Moisten the towel with water at a temperature of 105°F

15. A nurse is caring for a female client with a fractured arm. How should the nurse care for the client's hair? Select all that apply.

    a. Brush the hair for a longer time

    b. Tie the hair into a bun

    c. Use a wide-tooth comb

    d. Brush the hair slowly and carefully

    e. Start combing the hair from the crown

16. A nurse is assisting a client in cleaning his eyeglasses. Arrange the tasks in the most likely sequence in which the nurse should perform them when caring for the client's eyeglasses.

    a. Wash the lenses with soap or detergent

    b. Rinse with running tap water

    c. Hold the eyeglasses by the nose or ear braces

    d. Run tepid water over both sides of the lenses

    e. Dry with a clean, soft cloth such as a handkerchief

17. A client who has just started wearing contact lenses needs some help in removing them. Arrange the tasks in the most likely sequence in which the nurse should perform them when removing the client's contact lenses.

a. Remove the lenses using the thumb and forefinger

b. Place a towel on the client's chest

c. Compresses the lid margins together

d. Elevate the client's head

e. Move the contact lens from the cornea to the sclera

18. The nurse, while giving a towel bath, has to prefold and moisten the towel with approximately one half gallon of water, which is approximately _____ L of water.

a. 2

b. 1.5

c. 2.5

d. 1

CHAPTER 18

Comfort, Rest, and Sleep

SECTION I: LEARNING OBJECTIVES

- Differentiate between comfort, rest, and sleep.
- Describe four ways to modify the client environment to promote comfort, rest, and sleep.
- List four standard furnishings in each client room.
- State at least five functions of sleep.
- Describe the two phases of sleep and their differences.
- Describe the general trend in sleep requirements as a person ages.
- Name 10 factors that affect sleep.
- List four categories of drugs that affect sleep.
- Name four techniques for assessing sleep patterns.
- Describe four categories of sleep disorders.
- Discuss at least five techniques for promoting sleep.
- Name two nursing measures that promote relaxation.
- Discuss unique characteristics of sleep among older adults.

SECTION II: ASSESSING YOUR UNDERSTANDING

ACTIVITY A *Fill in the blanks.*

1. _____ is the ability to maintain stable body temperature.

2. The rapid eye movement (REM) phase of sleep is referred to as _____ sleep.

3. _____ are conditions associated with activities that cause arousal or partial arousal usually during transitions in non-REM (NREM) periods of sleep.

4. _____ are a class of drugs that excite structures in the brain and causes wakefulness.

5. _____ means difficulty falling asleep, awakening frequently during the night, or awakening early.

6. _____ is a technique for suppressing melatonin by stimulating light receptors in the eye and is prescribed for seasonal affective disorder.

7. _____ refers to the waking state characterized by reduced activity and mental stimulation.

8. The onset of disorientation as the sun sets is referred to as _____ syndrome.

9. _____ is a sleep disorder characterized by feeling sleepy despite getting normal sleep.

Activity B *Consider the following figures.*

Awake:
low-voltage, fast

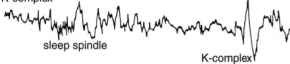

Awake eyes closed:
alpha-waves, 8–12 cps

NREM:
Stage 1:
theta-waves, 3–7 cps

Stage 2:
sleep spindles, 12–14 cps;
K-complex

sleep spindle

K-complex

Stages 3 and 4:
delta-waves, 0.5–2 cps

REM:
low-voltage mixed frequency
sawtoothed waves

sawtooth

1. Identify the figure.

_____

_____

_____

2. Explain the phases of sleep.

_____

_____

_____

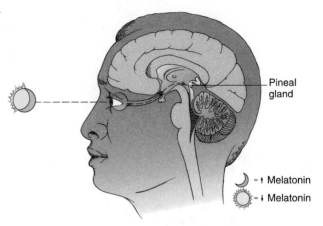

Pineal gland

☾ = ↑ Melatonin

☀ = ↓ Melatonin

3. Identify the figure.

_____

_____

_____

4. Explain the role of phototherapy in the sleep–wake cycle.

_____

_____

_____

Activity C *Match the types of parasomnias in column A with their descriptions in column B.*

Column A

___ **1.** Nocturnal enuresis

___ **2.** Somnambulism

___ **3.** Bruxism

___ **4.** Restless legs syndrome

Column B

A. Condition in which the individual walks in his or her sleep

B. Condition in which the individual grinds his or her teeth during sleep

C. Movement, typically in the legs, to relieve disturbing skin sensations

D. Also known as bed-wetting

Activity D *Briefly answer the following.*

1. What are the functions of sleep?

_____

_____

_____

2. What is progressive relaxation?

_____

_____

_____

3. What are the factors that affect sleep?

_____

_____

_____

4. What is nocturnal polysomnography?

_____

_____

_____

5. What is seasonal affective disorder?

_____

_____

_____

Activity E _Use the clues to complete the crossword puzzle._

Across

1. Unintentional sleep lasting 20 to 30 seconds
2. Sudden loss of muscle tone triggered by an emotional change such as happiness or anger
3. Grinding of the teeth

Down

4. Syndrome characterized by early-morning confusion associated with inadequate sleep or the effects of sedative and hypnotic medications
5. Hormones that induce drowsiness and sleep
6. Decreased cellular oxygenation

SECTION III: APPLYING YOUR KNOWLEDGE

Activity F *During the apneic or hypopneic periods of sleep apnea, ventilation decreases and blood oxygenation decreases. The accumulation of carbon dioxide and the decrease in oxygen cause brief periods of awakening throughout the night. This disturbs the normal transitions and periods of NREM and REM sleep. Answer the following questions, which involve the nurse's role in the physical assessment of clients.*

A client is admitted to the health care facility with a diagnosis of sleep apnea. The nurse understands that the condition can be life-threatening at times.

1. What are the risks associated with sleep apnea?

   _____

   _____

   _____

2. What nursing interventions should the nurse implement to promote sleep in the client?

   _____

   _____

   _____

SECTION IV: PRACTICING FOR NCLEX

Activity G *Answer the following questions.*

1. A nurse is caring for a client diagnosed with somnambulism. Which of the following activities should the nurse include in the plan of care for this client?
   a. Keep the client restrained
   b. Lock the stair gates and doors
   c. Keep a call bell within reach of the client
   d. Administer sedatives if prescribed

2. A client is admitted to the health care facility after getting a plaster cast put on a fractured tibia. Which of the following accessories of the bed should the nurse use to provide comfort to the fractured leg?
   a. Mattress
   b. Blanket
   c. Pillows
   d. Headboard

3. During the process of cardiopulmonary resuscitation (CPR), which of the following furnishings of the client's room may help in giving effective CPR?
   a. Over-the-bed table
   b. Side stand
   c. Bedside chair
   d. Headboard

4. A nurse is caring for a client who is bedridden as a result of a spinal cord injury. Which of the following interventions should the nurse implement to keep the client's skin intact?
   a. Place an extra draw sheet
   b. Provide extra pillows
   c. Place a mattress overlay
   d. Provide a soft mattress

5. A nurse finds that a client with leg ulcers has swelling resulting from infection. Which of the following should be the first nursing intervention to treat swelling?
   a. Elevate the limb with pillows
   b. Immobilize the affected limb
   c. Change the wound dressing
   d. Restrict fluid intake

6. What nursing intervention should a nurse perform for a client who has been diagnosed with urinary incontinence to prevent the frequent changing of bed linens?
   a. Restricting the amount of fluid intake by the client
   b. Placing an absorbent pad between the client and the bottom sheet
   c. Providing an extra bottom sheet to the client
   d. Adding an extra draw sheet on the bed of the client

7. A nurse is examining the mastectomy site in a female client a week after breast surgery. Which of the following nursing interventions is the most appropriate to maintain the dignity of the client?
   a. Provide an explanation for the procedure
   b. Draw the privacy curtain around the client
   c. Place the client in a comfortable position
   d. Use soft strokes when palpating the site

8. What intervention should the nurse perform to prevent hypoxia in a client with sleep apnea?

   a. Provide a special breathing mask
   b. Encourage physical exercises
   c. Provide milk before sleeping
   d. Provide a back massage before sleep

9. A client visits the health care facility with complaints of sleeplessness. During the interview, the client tells the nurse that he awakens early and then is unable to get any sleep. Which of the following nursing interventions would be appropriate for the client?

   a. Ask the client to join an exercise regimen
   b. Ask the client to engage in diversional activities
   c. Ask the client to avoid alcohol before sleeping
   d. Ask the client to avoid listening to stimulating music

10. A nurse is caring for a client who is unable to get proper sleep as a result of an increased frequency in urination. Which of the following interventions should the nurse implement to help the client?

   a. Administer diuretics in the morning
   b. Reduce the dose of diuretics in the evening
   c. Get a physician's order for catheterization
   d. Restrict fluid intake for the client

11. A nurse is preparing a discharge teaching for a client with narcolepsy. Which of the following activities should the nurse suggest the client avoid?

   a. Driving motor vehicles
   b. Performing moderate exercise
   c. Watching television before sleep
   d. Practicing relaxation techniques

12. A client who visits the health care center complains to the nurse that lately he has been lacking energy when he is awake; however, his appetite has increased, accompanied by a craving for sweets, which has led to weight gain. The client has noticed that these symptoms begin during darker winter months and disappear as daylight hours increase in the spring. Which of the following therapies would be suitable for this client?

   a. Tranquilizers
   b. Relaxation
   c. Back massage
   d. Phototherapy

13. A client is admitted to the health care facility for an angiography that has been scheduled for the next day. The client tells the nurse that he is unable to sleep because the place is new to him. What appropriate nursing diagnosis should the nurse record for this client?

   a. Impaired bed mobility
   b. Disturbed sleep pattern
   c. Relocation stress syndrome
   d. Impaired gas exchange

14. A nurse is providing a back massage to a client to facilitate relaxation. Which of the following should the nurse keep in mind when giving a back massage?

   a. Perform circular strokes
   b. Omit stimulating strokes
   c. Ask the client to relax
   d. Perform firm strokes

15. An elderly client is admitted to the health care unit with insomnia. Which of the following nursing interventions should the nurse implement to promote sleep in the client? Select all that apply.

   a. Promote physical exercise
   b. Administer sedatives as prescribed
   c. Provide milk before sleeping
   d. Provide a warmer environment
   e. Encourage relaxation techniques

16. A client visits his primary health care facility with complaints of difficulty in falling asleep. As a part of health education, which of the following food items should the nurse tell the client to avoid before bedtime? Select all that apply.

   a. Coffee
   b. Cola
   c. Chocolate
   d. Fish
   e. Legumes

CHAPTER 19

Safety

SECTION I: LEARNING OBJECTIVES

- Give an example of one common injury that predominates during each developmental stage (infancy through older adulthood).
- Name six injuries that result from environmental hazards.
- Identify at least two methods for reducing latex sensitization.
- List four areas of responsibility incorporated into most fire plans.
- Describe the indications for using each class of fire extinguishers.
- Discuss five measures for preventing burns.
- Name three common causes of asphyxiation.
- Discuss two methods for preventing drowning.
- Explain why humans are susceptible to electrical shock.
- Discuss three methods for preventing electrical shock.
- Name at least six common substances associated with poisonings.
- Discuss four methods for preventing poisonings.
- Discuss the benefits and risks of using physical restraints.
- Explain the basis for enacting restraint legislation and JCAHO accreditation standards.
- Differentiate between a restraint and a restraint alternative.
- Give at least four criteria for applying a physical restraint.
- Describe two areas of concern during an accident.
- Explain why older adults are prone to falling.

SECTION II: ASSESSING YOUR UNDERSTANDING

Activity A *Fill in the blanks.*

1. A(n) _____ burn is a skin injury caused by flames, hot liquids, or steam and is the most common form of burn.

2. _____ is the inability to breathe and results from airway obstruction, drowning, or inhalation of noxious gases such as smoke or carbon monoxide.

3. _____ is a harmless distribution of low-amperage electricity over a large area of the body.

4. _____ are used to restrict a person's freedom of movement, physical activity, or normal access to his or her body.

5. _____ dermatitis refers to a delayed localized skin reaction that occurs within 6 to 48 hours and lasts several days.

6. A(n) _____ is a substance that facilitates the flow of electrical current.

7. _____ is a plan or set of steps to follow when implementing an intervention.

8. _____ refers to the loss of bone mass, which increases the risk for fractures, especially in older women.

9. A _____ diverts leaking electrical energy to the earth.

10. _____ is low-voltage but high-amperage electricity.

Activity B *Consider the following figures.*

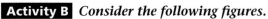

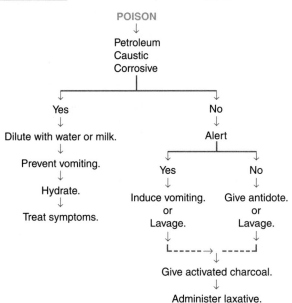

POISON
↓
Petroleum
Caustic
Corrosive

Yes   No
↓   ↓
Dilute with water or milk.   Alert
↓
Prevent vomiting.   Yes   No
↓   ↓   ↓
Hydrate.   Induce vomiting.   Give antidote.
↓   or   or
Treat symptoms.   Lavage.   Lavage.
↓   ↓
Give activated charcoal.
↓
Administer laxative.

1. Identify the figure.

_____

_____

_____

2. Explain the management of accidental poisoning.

_____

_____

_____

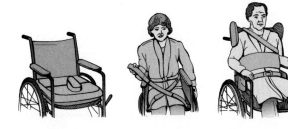

3. Identify the figure.

_____

_____

_____

4. Differentiate between restraints and restraint alternatives.

_____

_____

_____

Activity C *Match the type of extinguisher in column A with the type of substances it is used for in column B.*

Column A   **Column B**

____ **1.** Class A   **A.** Gasoline, oil, paint, grease and other flammable liquids

____ **2.** Class B

____ **3.** Class C   **B.** Electrical fires

____ **4.** Class ABC   **C.** Fires of any kind

               D. Burning paper, wood, cloth

Activity D *Presented here, in random order, are steps occurring during fire management. Write the correct sequence in the boxes provided.*

1. Rescue

2. Confine the fire

3. Alarm

4. Extinguish

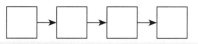

Presented here, in random order, are steps occurring during the management of accidental poisoning resulting from the consumption of sedatives. Write the correct sequence in the boxes provided.

1. Check for vital signs

2. Administer laxatives

3. Give activated charcoal

4. Induce vomiting

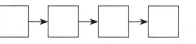

Activity E *Briefly answer the following.*

1. What are the types of latex reaction?

_____

_____

_____

2. What are the methods used to prevent thermal burns?

_____

_____

_____

3. What is meant by carbon monoxide poisoning?

_____

_____

_____

4. What measure should be practiced to prevent drowning?

_____

_____

_____

5. What is meant by restraint alternatives?

_____

_____

_____

Activity F   _Use the clues to complete the crossword puzzle._

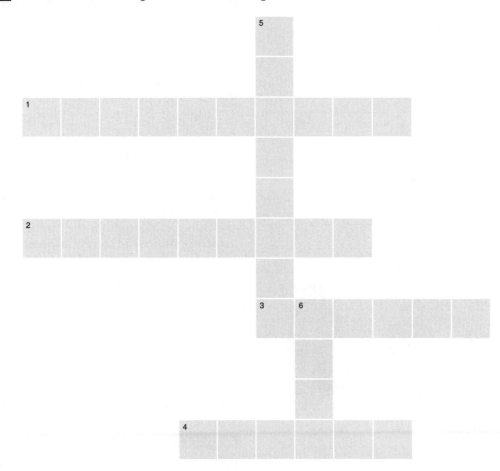

Across

1. An exaggerated fear of falling
2. Injury caused by the ingestion, inhalation, or absorption of a toxic substance
3. It diverts leaking electrical energy to the earth
4. Prevention of accidents or unintentional injuries

Down

5. Condition in which fluid occupies the airway and interferes with ventilation
6. Acronym to identify the basic steps to take when managing a fire

SECTION III: APPLYING YOUR KNOWLEDGE

Activity G *In health care agencies, fall prevention measures may include the use of physical and chemical restraints, which are methods of restricting a person's freedom of movement, physical activity, or normal access to his or her body. The use of restraints, however, is closely regulated. Answer the following questions, which involve the nurse's role in the use of restraints.*

A nurse is caring for an elderly client who is confused but has a steady gait. Repeatedly, the client tries to get out of the room. The nurse plans to restrain the client to prevent him from walking off the premises.

1. What kind of alternative restraint should the nurse use on the client?

_____

_____

_____

2. What are the disadvantages of conventional restraints?

_____

_____

_____

SECTION IV: PRACTICING FOR NCLEX

Activity H *Answer the following questions.*

1. A nurse is planning a discharge teaching for an elderly client with cognitive impairment. Which of the following interventions should the nurse adopt to ensure that the client does not take an accidental overdose of medicines?

a. Write the medication order on a piece of paper

b. Prefill separate containers for the medicines

c. Instruct the client to see the blister pack

d. Explain the drug regimen to the client

2. A 4-year-old child with accidental poisoning resulting from the consumption of sedative medications is brought to the health care facility. Which of the following actions should be the first priority of the nurse?

a. Take a detailed history

b. Induce vomiting in the child

c. Assess breathing and cardiac function

d. Give gastric lavage

3. A nurse finds that a client in the psychiatric nursing unit is looking frightened and expresses that he is feeling out of control. Which of the following nursing interventions is the most appropriate?

a. Restrain the client on the bed

b. Isolate the client in a time-out room

c. Administer the prescribed anti-anxiety medication

d. Move the client into a quiet room and talk to him

4. A nurse is preparing a discharge teaching for a 10-month-old baby with his mother. Which of the following teachings should the nurse include to prevent accidental falls in the infant?

a. Educate the parents to restrain the infant in automobiles

b. Avoid making the baby sit on a chair or bed

c. Keep the baby restrained while feeding

d. Prevent the baby from moving around

5. A nurse is providing health education in a pediatric clinic about the prevention of accidental poisoning in toddlers. Which of the following activities should the nurse encourage in parents?

a. Avoid keeping any cleaning solutions at home

b. Educate kids about the consequences of poisoning

c. Label poisonous substances

d. Keep cleaning solutions locked

6. A nurse is caring for a client who is restrained as a result of a psychiatric condition. The nurse prepares a plan of care for the client. Which of the following nursing diagnoses should be a priority in the client?

   a. Impaired mobility

   b. Risk for injury

   c. Impaired sensory perception

   d. Altered consciousness

7. A nurse-in-charge is educating team members about electrical safety and the prevention of electrical hazards in the nursing unit. Which of the following safety factors should the nurse emphasize the most?

   a. Unplug the equipment after use

   b. Put electrical cords under the carpet

   c. Use grounded equipment

   d. Avoid operating devices with wet hands

8. A toddler is admitted to the health care facility for a diagnostic test scheduled the next day. Which of the following nursing activities should be the highest priority for the nurse?

   a. Protect the toddler from injury

   b. Befriend the toddler for confidence

   c. Adapt the toddler to hospital routines

   d. Prepare for the diagnostic test

9. A nurse is caring for an elderly, disoriented client who has been restrained. On reassessment, the nurse finds that the client has improved, but the restraint order is for another 2 hours. Which of the following nursing interventions is the most appropriate action?

   a. Wait for the physician to inspect the client and revise the order

   b. Remove the restraint, even if the order has not expired

   c. Continue the restraint until the order has expired

   d. Loosen the restraint to allow limited movement

10. An industrial health nurse is preparing a health education class about the management of carbon monoxide poisoning. Which of the following interventions are appropriate to manage carbon monoxide poisoning? Select all that apply.

    a. Remove the person from the site.

    b. Check for vital signs.

    c. Administer oxygen inhalation.

    d. Keep the doors and windows closed.

    e. Reorient the client.

11. Upon entering a client's room, a nurse finds that there is an outbreak of fire from an electrical point. Which of the following nursing actions should be the highest priority?

    a. Call for the electrician

    b. Raise the alarm for help

    c. Extinguish the fire

    d. Evacuate the client

12. A nurse gets an order to restrain a client for 2 hours with a restraint alternative. Which of the following is a restraint alternative? Select all that apply.

    a. Tilt wedges

    b. Vest restraint

    c. Seat belts with Velcro

    d. Harnesses with buckles

    e. Elbow restraints

13. A nurse is preparing discharge teaching for a 5-year-old client admitted with accidental drowning. Which of the following health teachings should be included for the parents to prevent further incidences of drowning? Select all that apply.

    a. Never let the child swim alone

    b. Provide life jackets when swimming

    c. Let the child swim with his friends

    d. Keep the swimming pool fenced

    e. Let the child swim alone to gain confidence

14. A nurse is caring for a client who is repeatedly trying to take out the endotracheal tube that facilitates breathing. Which of the following would be an appropriate action taken by the nurse to prevent the client from removing the endotracheal tube?

    a. Apply elbow restraints to the client

    b. Tell a family member to sit with the client

    c. Take a restraint order from a physician by telephone

    d. Apply waist restraints to the client

15. A 10-year-old boy is brought to the primary health center with wounds on his knees. Which of the following could be the possible cause of the injury in the child?

    a. Play-related activities

    b. Automobile accident

    c. A fall from a bed

    d. A fall down the stairs

16. A nurse is caring for a client who develops contact dermatitis on exposure to latex. Which of the following interventions should the nurse implement to protect the client from latex exposure? Select all that apply.

    a. Attach an allergy-alert ID bracelet to the client

    b. Stock the client's room with latex-free equipment

    c. Communicate with other personnel to use non-latex equipment

    d. Wash hands before wearing gloves to provide care to the client

    e. Instruct the client to wash the area in contact with latex immediately

17. An empty client room has caught fire. The nurse takes all measures according to the fire plan of the health care facility. The nurse finds that the smoke is escaping from the room into the corridors. Which of the following measures should the nurse implement to prevent smoke from escaping the room?

    a. Close the door of the room on fire

    b. Place a moist blanket at the thresholds of the doors

    c. Switch on the fans in the corridors to spread the smoke

    d. Wait for the firemen to come and handle it

18. A nurse is planning a discharge teaching for an elderly client. Which of the following measures should the nurse include in her teaching to prevent falls in the client?

    a. Wear slippers at home

    b. Walk with a supporting cane

    c. Call for assistance to ambulate

    d. Avoid keeping area rugs

CHAPTER 20

Pain Management

SECTION I: LEARNING OBJECTIVES

- Give a general definition of pain.
- List four phases in the pain process.
- Explain the difference between pain perception, pain threshold, and pain tolerance.
- Describe the gate–control theory of pain transmission.
- Discuss how endogenous opioids reduce pain transmission.
- Name at least five types of pain.
- Give at least three characteristics that differentiate acute pain from chronic pain.
- List five components of a basic pain assessment.
- Name four common pain intensity assessment tools that nurses use.
- Identify at least three occasions when it is essential to perform a pain assessment and document assessment findings.
- Name four physiologic mechanisms for managing pain.
- Give three categories of drugs used alone or in combination to manage pain.
- Identify two surgical procedures used when other methods of pain management are ineffective.
- List at least five non-drug, non-surgical methods for managing pain.
- Discuss the most common reason why clients request frequent administrations of pain-relieving drugs.
- Define addiction.
- Discuss how addiction affects pain management.
- Define placebo and explain the basis for its positive effect.

SECTION II: ASSESSING YOUR UNDERSTANDING

Activity A *Fill in the blanks.*

1. _____ assessment is the fifth vital sign usually associated with disease or injury that causes physical discomfort.

2. _____ is the last phase of pain impulse transmission in which the brain interacts with the spinal nerves to alter the pain experience.

3. _____ pain lasts longer than 6 months.

4. _____ prevents sensory impulses from entering the spinal cord and traveling to the brain.

5. With _____, a client learns to control or alter a physiologic phenomenon as an adjunct to traditional pain management.

6. _____ is the intentional diversion of attention to switch the person's focus from an unpleasant sensory experience to one that is neutral.

7. _____ refers to the conversion of chemical information at the cellular level into electrical impulses that move toward the spinal cord.

8. _____ are a type of sensory nerve receptor activated by noxious stimuli located in the skin, bones, joints, muscles, and internal organs.

9. _____ drugs relieve pain by altering neurotransmission peripherally at the site of injury.

10. _____ is a pain management technique in which long, thin needles are inserted into the client's skin.

Activity B *Consider the following figure.*

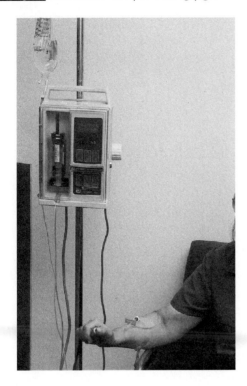

1. Identify the image.

_____

_____

_____

2. What are the advantages of this mechanism?

_____

_____

Activity C *Match the pain management techniques in column A with their descriptions in column B.*

Column A

____ 1. Thermal therapy

____ 2. Transcutaneous electrical nerve stimulation (TENS)

Column B

A. Passing of an electrical stimulus through tiny needles inserted within the soft tissue

B. Compression of tissues to reduce pain

____ 3. Acupressure

____ 4. Percutaneous electrical nerve stimulation (PENS)

____ 5. Hypnosis

C. Applications of hot or cold packs on the affected body part

D. Initiating a person to enter a trancelike state resulting in an alteration in perception and memory

E. Delivers bursts of electricity to the skin and underlying nerves

Activity D *Presented here, in random order, are the four phases in which people experience pain. Write the correct sequence in the boxes provided.*

1. Modulation

2. Transmission

3. Transduction

4. Perception

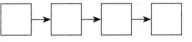

Activity E *Briefly answer the following.*

1. How does transmission of pain occur?

_____

_____

_____

2. What is acute pain?

_____

_____

_____

3. What is transduction and when does it begin?

_____

_____

_____

4. In what type of research trials has PENS been successful on clients?

_____

_____

_____

5. How can placebos help a client to relieve pain?

_____

_____

_____

6. What are the factors that influence pain tolerance in clients?

_____

_____

_____

Activity F _Use the clues to complete the crossword puzzle._

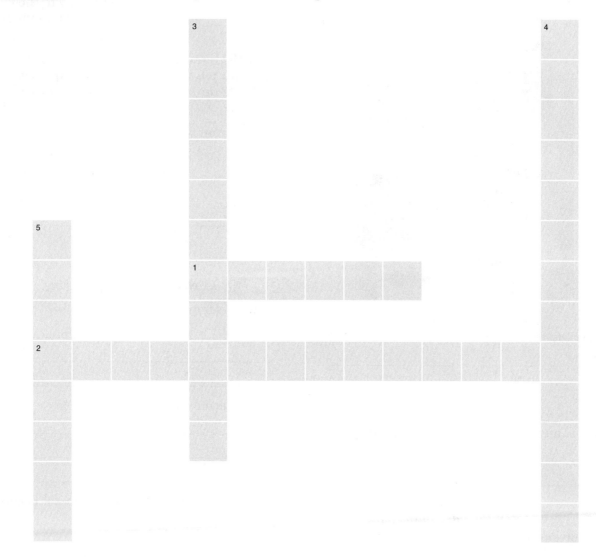

Across

1. It is used in chemical rhizotomy
2. It is one of the newest categories of non-opioid drugs

Down

3. They are a type of sensory nerve receptor activated by noxious stimuli
4. It is the most widely used anticonvulsant
5. They are an inactive substance prescribed as a substitute for an analgesic drug

SECTION III: APPLYING YOUR KNOWLEDGE

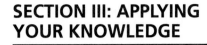 **Activity G** *When caring for clients in pain, the most important nursing process is pain assessment. Nurses should thoroughly document the client's pain to gather objective data about a client. Answer the following questions, which involve the nurse's role in the pain assessment of clients.*

A nurse is caring for an elderly client at the health care facility. During the pain assessment, the nurse asks the client about her pain and the names and dosages of pain medicine that the client has been taking. The client informs the nurse that she is in great pain and is unable to recollect the name and dosage of her medication.

1. What interventions should the nurse follow when conducting pain assessments?

   _____

   _____

   _____

2. What kinds of behavioral signs should the nurse observe when assessing pain in clients?

   _____

   _____

   _____

SECTION IV: PRACTICING FOR NCLEX

Activity H *Answer the following questions.*

1. Per the direction of the physician, the nurse needs to administer pain medication to an elderly client, who complains of acute abdominal pain. What intervention should the nurse follow for effective absorption of the medication?
   a. Rectal route
   b. Oral route
   c. Nasal route
   d. Intramuscular route

2. A nurse is administering a prescribed non-opioid drug to a client. A non-opioid will be most effective for pain caused by which of the following?
   a. Headache
   b. Injury
   c. Weak muscles
   d. Inflammation

3. A physician directs a nurse to use an EMG machine on an elderly client. Which of the following is the function of an EMG machine?
   a. To produce signals correlating with the person's heart rate, skin temperature, or muscle tension
   b. To produce signals correlating with the person's pain
   c. To produce signals correlating with the person's age and intramuscular tension
   d. To produce signals correlating with the person's age and body mass index

4. A nurse is conducting the initial interview for a client who has been admitted to the health care facility with chronic back pain. What questions related to pain assessment should the nurse ask during the interview?
   a. "Do you ever take pain medications in the morning?"
   b. "What are the names and dosages of pain medicine you take?"
   c. "Does your daily diet contain any calcium supplements?"
   d. "Are you able to do strenuous activities despite the pain?"

5. A nurse is caring for a client with complaints of severe backache who has been prescribed TENS as a pain management technique. The nurse should know which of the following candidates are contraindicated and should seek medical advice before opting for TENS. Select all that apply.
   a. Clients involved in sports activities
   b. Clients who are pregnant
   c. Clients with cardiac pacemakers
   d. Clients prone to irregular heartbeats
   e. Clients who are young adults

6. A client with acute pain in the spinal cord has been prescribed an intraspinal analgesia. How much intraspinal analgesia should the nurse administer to the client?

   a. Several times a day or as a continuous low-dose infusion

   b. Once a day with high-dose infusion

   c. Twice a day with low-dose infusion

   d. Once in 6 months with continuous low-dose infusion

7. A nurse is caring for a 3-year-old client who is in pain. Which of the following pain scales should the nurse use to assess this client?

   a. Numeric scale

   b. Word scale

   c. Linear scale

   d. Faces scale

8. A nurse is caring for an elderly client who has been complaining of a back pain for the past 8 months. The client's daughter informs the nurse that lately her mother gets angry over minor issues. Which of the following are common reactions of persons associated with clients in chronic pain? Select all that apply.

   a. They suggest that the pain has a psychological basis

   b. They suggest that the client is addicted to pain medication

   c. They say that the client uses drugs as a crutch

   d. They say that they pay close attention to the client's concerns

   e. They say they are eager to hear about the client's pain

9. A client whose left limb has been amputated after an accident 2 months earlier complains to the nurse that he experiences a burning, itching, and deep pain in the amputated limb. What kind of pain is the client experiencing?

   a. Somatic pain

   b. Chronic pain

   c. Acute pain

   d. Neuropathic pain

10. A nurse is caring for a client with acute abdominal pain. The physician directs the nurse to administer dosages of meperidine. What are the different ways in which the nurse can administer meperidine to the client? Select all that apply.

    a. Oral route

    b. Sublingual route

    c. Rectal route

    d. Intramuscular route

    e. Transdermal route

11. A client is taking antidepressant drugs prescribed by the physician. What should be the desired effect of the antidepressant drug on the client?

    a. Increase the norepinephrine and serotonin levels

    b. Regulate the inhibitory neurotransmitter gamma-aminobutyric acid

    c. Block the release of substance P and other inflammatory chemicals

    d. Stimulate the body of the client to release endogenous opioids

12. A nurse is caring for a client who has been prescribed several drugs to treat chronic back pain. The client asks for non-drug and non-surgical interventions in pain management. Which of the following are non-drug and non-surgical interventions in pain management? Select all that apply.

    a. Massage

    b. Cordotomy

    c. Meditation

    d. Hypnosis

    e. Acupressure

13. An elderly client is being treated for pain in the joints for several months. Initially, the client used to obtain some relief. Now, however, the client tells the nurse that despite taking the prescribed medicine, the pain continues to persist. Which could be the most accurate reason for the pain to continue despite the medication?

    a. The client's body may have developed a drug tolerance to the prescribed dose

    b. The physician may have prescribed a lower dosage

    c. The nurse may have administered lower levels of the prescribed drug

    d. The client's body may be absorbing the drug quickly

14. A nurse is caring for a client with under-treated pain. The client complains that his bowel motility has reduced considerably. What other autonomic nervous system responses should the nurse observe in a client with undertreated pain?
    a. Dilated pupils
    b. Dehydration
    c. Reduced glucose level
    d. Convulsions

15. A nurse is caring for a client who has developed somatic pain after a road accident. Which of the following leads to somatic pain?
    a. Injury to muscles, tendons, and joints
    b. Irritation to the dermis and epidermis
    c. Traumatic injury to the head and neck
    d. Effect of opioids and opiate analgesics

16. A client with acute upper abdominal pain has been admitted in the health care facility. Per JCAHO's pain assessment standards, which of the following is a nursing intervention when caring for this client?
    a. Assess the client's pain after checking the medical history
    b. Assess the client's pain once per shift
    c. Assess the client's pain and refer elsewhere
    d. Assess the client's pain on an hourly basis

17. After being administered a dosage of codeine sulfate for his knee pain, an elderly man complains of an uneasy sensation. What other symptoms should the nurse note that the client could experience after taking opioid drugs? Select all that apply.
    a. Sedation
    b. Nausea
    c. Diarrhea
    d. Respiratory depression
    e. Dilated pupils

18. A nurse is assessing a client with acute pain. Which of the following points should the nurse document when assessing the client?
    a. The client's discomfort has lasted longer than 6 months
    b. The client's discomfort originates at the skin level
    c. The client's discomfort reduces gradually with medicine
    d. The client is not showing autonomic nervous system responses

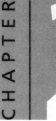
Oxygenation

SECTION I: LEARNING OBJECTIVES

- Explain the difference between ventilation and respiration.
- Differentiate between external and internal respiration.
- Name two methods for assessing the oxygenation status of clients at the bedside.
- List at least five signs of inadequate oxygenation.
- Name two nursing interventions that can be used to improve ventilation and oxygenation.
- Identify four items that may be needed when providing oxygen therapy.
- Name four sources of supplemental oxygen.
- List five common oxygen delivery devices.
- Discuss two hazards related to the administration of oxygen.
- Describe two additional therapeutic techniques that relate to oxygenation.
- Discuss at least two facts concerning oxygenation that affect the care of older adults.

SECTION II: ASSESSING YOUR UNDERSTANDING

Activity A *Fill in the blanks.*

1. _____ results from pressure changes within the thoracic cavity produced by the contraction and relaxation of respiratory muscles.

2. _____ means insufficient oxygen within arterial blood.

3. The _____ position allows room for maximum vertical and lateral chest expansion and provides comfort while resting or sleeping.

4. _____ breathing, which involves taking in a large volume of air, fills alveoli to a greater capacity, thus improving gas exchange.

5. A(n) _____ is a gauge used to regulate the amount of oxygen delivered to the client and is attached to the oxygen source.

6. A(n) _____ is a device that produces small water droplets and is used during oxygen administration.

7. A(n) _____ mask mixes a precise amount of oxygen and atmospheric air.

8. A(n) _____ collar delivers oxygen near an artificial opening in the neck.

9. As a client grows older, the chest walls become stiffer as a result of _____ of the intercostal muscles.

10. During _____, the dome-shaped diaphragm contracts and moves downward in the thorax.

Activity B *Consider the following figure.*

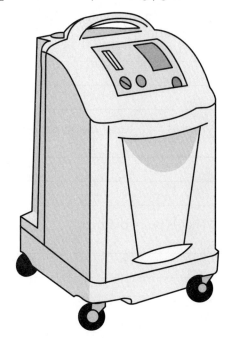

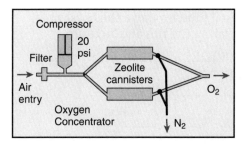

1. Identify the figure.

_____

_____

_____

2. What are the advantages of this equipment?

_____

_____

_____

Activity C *Match the terms related to oxygenation in column A with their description in column B.*

Column A

____ 1. Oxygen analyzer

____ 2. Nasal cannula

____ 3. Partial rebreather mask

____ 4. Pursed-lip breathing

____ 5. Incentive spirometry

Column B

A. Hollow tube with half-inch prongs placed into the client's nostrils

B. Oxygen delivery device through which a client inhales a mixture of atmospheric air, oxygen from its source, and oxygen contained within a reservoir bag

C. A technique for deep breathing, using a calibrated device

D. Measures the percentage of oxygen delivered to the client

E. A form of controlled ventilation in which the client consciously prolongs the expiration phase of breathing

Activity D *Presented here, in random order, are steps occurring during ventilation. Write the correct sequence in the boxes provided.*

1. The thoracic cavity expands.

2. Air is pulled in through the nose, filling the lungs.

3. The intercostal muscles move the chest outward by elevating the ribs and sternum.

4. Pressure within the lungs falls below pressure in the atmosphere.

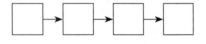

Activity E *Briefly answer the following.*

1. How does a nurse physically assess a client for oxygenation?

_____

_____

_____

2. What is an arterial blood gas assessment?

_____

_____

_____

3. What is pulse oximetry?

_____

_____

_____

4. What is oxygen therapy?

_____

_____

_____

5. What are the disadvantages of an oxygen concentrator?

_____

_____

_____

6. What is a non-breather mask?

_____

_____

_____

Activity F *Use the clues to complete the crossword puzzle.*

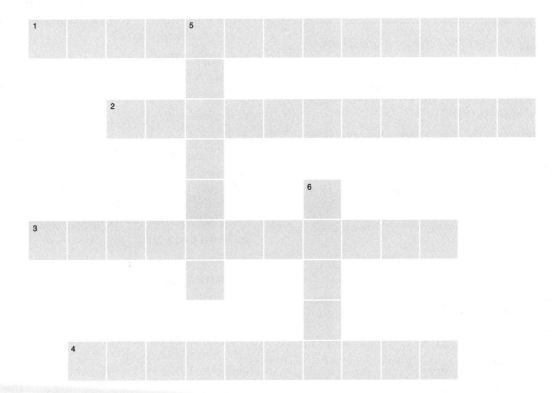

Across

1. A type of breathing that promotes the use of the diaphragm rather than the upper chest
2. Excessive levels of carbon dioxide in the blood
3. Exchange of carbon dioxide and oxygen
4. The process of breathing out

Down

5. Inadequate oxygen at the cellular level
6. Inserted into a surgically created opening before transtracheal oxygen is used

SECTION III: APPLYING YOUR KNOWLEDGE

Activity G *Many factors affect ventilation and, subsequently, respiration. Positioning and teaching breathing techniques are two nursing interventions frequently used to promote oxygenation. Answer the questions related to nursing intervention to promote oxygenation.*

A nurse is caring for a client who is brought to the health care facility with breathing difficulty. The client is diagnosed to have hypoxia.

1. In what position should the nurse place the client to promote better breathing?

   _____

   _____

   _____

2. What breathing techniques could the nurse teach the client to ensure efficient breathing?

   _____

   _____

   _____

SECTION IV: PRACTICING FOR NCLEX

Activity H *Answer the following questions.*

1. A client has been ordered an arterial blood gas test as part of assessing the quality of oxygenation. What is the arterial blood gas assessment test for?

   a. It measures the partial pressure of oxygen dissolved in plasma

   b. It measures the blood pressure of the client

   c. It monitors the oxygen saturation in the blood

   d. It monitors the level of consciousness of the client

2. A nurse is caring for a client who has been diagnosed with emphysema. Which of the following breathing techniques should the nurse teach the client to help him breathe more efficiently?

   a. Deep breathing

   b. Incentive spirometry

   c. Pursed-lip breathing

   d. Nasal strips

3. A client at the health care facility is provided with a liquid oxygen unit to keep the blood adequately saturated with oxygen. What should the nurse inform this client about the potential problems related to the liquid oxygen unit? Select all that apply.

   a. Frozen moisture may occlude the outlet

   b. It may leak during warm weather

   c. It is more expensive than other portable sources

   d. It produces an unpleasant odor

   e. Increases the electric bill

4. A nurse has been caring for a client who has been put on a ventilator in the ICU of the health care facility. Which of the following devices would help the nurse check whether the client is getting the prescribed amount of oxygen?

   a. Flowmeter

   b. Oxygen analyzer

   c. Humidifier

   d. Nasal cannula

5. Which of the following oxygen delivery devices should a nurse use for a client with facial burn injuries from a barbecue fire, who is also claustrophobic?

   a. Nasal cannula

   b. Face tent

   c. Tracheostomy collar

   d. T-piece

6. A nurse is caring for a 2-year-old client with symptoms of bronchitis. The nurse notices that the client is less active and is having difficulty breathing. Which device should the nurse use to deliver oxygen to the client to facilitate efficient breathing?

   a. Nasal catheter

   b. Oxygen tent

   c. Transtracheal catheter

   d. Continuous positive airway pressure (CPAP) mask

7. A nurse is caring for a client who is being administered oxygen through a transtracheal catheter. What precaution should the nurse take when cleaning the opening and the tube?

   a. Administer oxygen with a nasal cannula

   b. Administer oxygen with a Venturi mask

   c. Administer oxygen with a face tent

   d. Administer oxygen with a partial breather mask

8. A nurse is caring for a client with labored breathing. The client has been prescribed supplemental oxygen by the physician. When administering oxygen to the client, the nurse needs to be aware of oxygen toxicity. Which of the following situations could lead to oxygen toxicity in the client?

   a. Administration of 35% oxygen concentration for 24 hours

   b. Administration of 50% oxygen concentration for 36 hours

   c. Administration of 25% oxygen concentration for 48 hours

   d. Administration of 60% oxygen concentration for 48 hours

9. A nurse is treating a client for carbon monoxide poisoning. Which of the following oxygenation techniques could the nurse use to treat the client?

   a. Water-seal chest tube drainage

   b. Hyperbaric oxygen technique

   c. Liquid oxygen unit

   d. Oxygen concentrator

10. A 65-year-old client is being treated at the health care facility for a respiratory-related disorder. Which of the following should the nurse understand are age-related structural changes that affect the respiratory systems in older clients?

   a. Alveolar walls become thicker

   b. Lungs become more elastic

   c. More breathing from the mouth

   d. Chest walls become stiffer

11. A nurse is caring for a 45-year-old client at the health care facility with lowered respiratory function. What suggestion could the nurse make to improve the client's condition?

   a. Avoid strenuous exercise

   b. Use a nasal strip

   c. Drink fluids liberally

   d. Maintain proper skin care

12. A nurse is caring for an elderly client who requires administration of supplemental oxygen. The nurse uses a T-piece to administer oxygen to the client. What points should the nurse remember when using a T-piece to administer oxygen?

   a. It interferes with eating

   b. It creates a feeling of suffocation

   c. It delivers an inconsistent amount of oxygen

   d. It needs to be drained regularly

13. Arrange the following steps in the order that they occur during the process of expiration.

   a. Thoracic cavity decreases

   b. Intrathoracic pressure increases

   c. Respiratory muscles relax

   d. Lung tissue recoils

   e. Air exits the respiratory tract

14. Place the following steps in the order in which the nurse should teach a client to breathe using the pursed-lip technique.

   a. Contract the abdominal muscles

   b. Inhale slowly through the nose while counting to three

   c. Exhale through the pursed lips for a count of six or more

   d. Purse the lips as though to whistle

15. An oxygen tent is being used to administer oxygen to a 2.5-year-old client with bronchiolitis. What care should the nurse take when using an oxygen tent for the client? Select all that apply.

   a. Tuck the edges securely beneath the mattress

   b. Limit the opening of the zippered access port

   c. Monitor oxygen levels regularly with an analyzer

   d. Regulate the amount of oxygen delivered if inconsistent

   e. Provide proper skin care as a result of trapped moisture

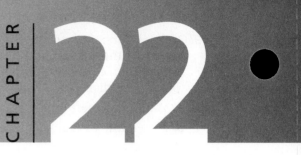

CHAPTER 22

Infection Control

SECTION I: LEARNING OBJECTIVES

- Explain the meaning of infectious diseases.
- Differentiate between infection and colonization.
- List five stages in the course of an infectious disease.
- Define infection control measures.
- Name two major techniques for infection control.
- Discuss situations in which nurses use standard precautions and transmission-based precautions.
- Describe the rationale for using airborne, droplet, and contact precautions.
- Explain the purpose of personal protective equipment.
- Discuss the rationale for removing personal protective equipment in a specific sequence after caring for a client with an infection.
- Explain how nurses perform double-bagging.
- List two psychological problems common among clients with infectious diseases.
- Provide at least three teaching suggestions for preventing infections.
- Discuss one unique characteristic of older adults in relation to infectious diseases.

SECTION II: ASSESSING YOUR UNDERSTANDING

Activity A *Fill in the blanks.*

1. _____ is a condition that results when microorganisms cause injury to a host.

2. _____ is a condition during which microorganisms are present, but the host does not manifest any signs or symptoms of infection.

3. Nurses should remove their _____ and wash their hands immediately before caring for another client.

4. _____ waste containers are emptied at the end of each shift.

5. Maintaining _____ skin is an excellent first-line defense against acquiring nosocomial infections.

6. The incidence of _____ infection in community-living elderly persons is twice that of the general population.

7. The use of standard precautions reduces the potential for transmitting _____ pathogens from moist body substances.

8. Symptoms of infections tend to be _____ among elderly clients.

9. Diseases spread from one person to another are also called _____ or communicable diseases.

10. _____ trash is refuse that will decompose naturally into less complex compounds.

Activity B *Consider the following figure.*

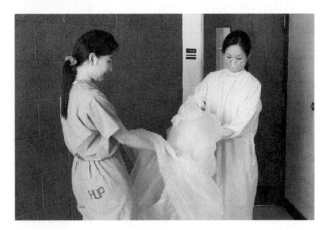

1. Identify the image.

   _____

   _____

   _____

2. What are the advantages of this technique?

   _____

   _____

   _____

Activity C *Match the stages of infectious diseases in column A with their characteristic in column B.*

Column A

_____ 1. Incubation period

_____ 2. Prodromal stage

_____ 3. Acute stage

_____ 4. Convalescent stage

Column B

A. Host overcomes the infectious agent

B. Symptoms become severe and specific

C. Initial symptoms are vague and non-specific

D. Infectious agent reproduces and exits host

Activity D *Presented here, in random order, are steps that occur during the removal of personal protective equipment worn by nurses. Write the correct sequence in the boxes provided.*

1. Roll up the gown and discard it in the waste container.

2. Remove the gown without touching the front side.

3. Fold the soiled side of the gown to the inside.

4. Remove the mask and other disposable face protection items.

5. Remove the gloves and discard them in a lined waste container.

6. Untie the waist closure if it is fastened at the front of the cover gown.

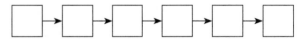

Activity E *Briefly answer the following.*

1. How can nurses promote social interaction for infectious clients?

   _____

   _____

   _____

2. Why are elderly clients more susceptible to infections?

   _____

   _____

   _____

3. What are the three types of transmission-based precautions?

   _____

   _____

   _____

4. What is meant by the terms *direct* and *indirect contact* in contact precautions?

   _____

   _____

   _____

5. Which items are included in personal protection equipment?

_____

_____

_____

6. Why are soiled dressings wrapped before being destroyed?

_____

_____

_____

Activity F _Use the clues to complete the crossword puzzle._

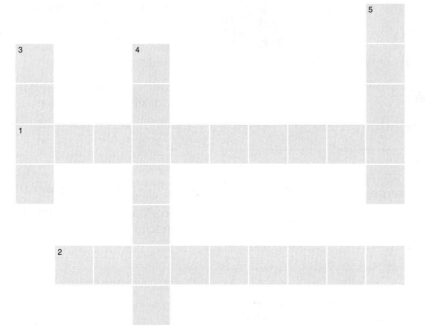

Across

1. Stage when the pathogen is destroyed and health is restored
2. An infectious disease common in residents of long-term care facilities

Down

3. Infectious diseases requiring both airborne and contact precautions
4. Precaution taken when client has rubella or influenza
5. Body substance that can transmit blood-borne pathogens

SECTION III: APPLYING YOUR KNOWLEDGE

Activity G *Infectious diseases spread from one person to another. Hence, prevention and proper infection control are the best ways to tackle infectious diseases. Answer the following questions, which involve a nurse's role in infection control.*

A nurse is caring for an elderly client with influenza at the health care facility. However, the client does not show any major symptoms of the infection. The client's family members have come to visit him at the health care facility because he is a long-term resident there.

1. What precautions should the nurse take to avoid the transmission of pathogens?

   _____

   _____

   _____

2. Why do symptoms of infections tend to be more subtle among elderly clients?

   _____

   _____

   _____

SECTION IV: PRACTICING FOR NCLEX

Activity H *Answer the following questions.*

1. A nurse is caring for an elderly client who has been prescribed an indwelling catheter. Which of the following measures should the nurse take to prevent urinary tract infections?
   a. Place the catheter tubing lower than the client's bladder
   b. Clean the client's urinary and rectal area
   c. Clean the indwelling catheter every week
   d. Bend the catheter tubing slightly toward the bladder

2. A client with pulmonary tuberculosis is returning to his private room from the X-ray department. Which of the following should the nurse do when the tuberculous client returns to his room?
   a. Cover the client's body with a second sheet on his return
   b. Line the edge of the client's bed with a clean sheet
   c. Spray the X-ray department with disinfectant after the client leaves
   d. Deposit the soiled linen in the linen hamper in the client's room

3. A nurse needs to collect contaminated material from the room of a client with pulmonary tuberculosis. Which of the following infection control measures should the nurse remember when double-bagging?
   a. Collect articles in a sturdy bag without contaminating the outside of the bag
   b. Place bulkier items in a trash bag and remove them from the room
   c. Place biodegradable trash in a plastic biohazard bag and destroy it in an incinerator
   d. Wear a non-sterile gown and spray disinfectant on the contaminated material

4. A nurse has finished cleaning the infectious warts of a client and needs to apply the prescribed medicine to the infected area. Which of the following precautions should the nurse take when caring for the client?
   a. Remove the contaminated cover gown before leaving the client's room
   b. Change gloves between tasks when caring for the client
   c. Wash hands thoroughly before leaving the client's room
   d. Make contact between two contaminated surfaces or two clean surfaces

5. A group of nurses are caring for victims of bioterrorism. Which of the following respirator masks should the nurses equip themselves when caring for victims of a bioterrorist attack?
   a. Atomizer
   b. N-95 respirator
   c. Drinker respirator
   d. Powered air-purifying respirator

6. A nurse needs to administer an intravenous drug to a client with chickenpox and the common cold. Which of the following precautions should the nurse adhere to before entering the client's room? Select all that apply.

   a. Standard

   b. Contact

   c. Airborne

   d. Droplet

   e. Basic

7. A nurse observes that a client with full-blown AIDS looks very frightened and refuses to meet anybody. Which of the following is the most appropriate nursing diagnosis for the client?

   a. Risk of infection

   b. Social isolation

   c. Ineffective protection

   d. Powerlessness

8. Two nurses are bagging contaminated material from the room of a client per the double-bagging method. Which of the following actions is performed during double-bagging?

   a. Biodegradable waste is collected in two plastic bags

   b. Contaminated material is disposed of in two separate bags

   c. One bag of contaminated items is placed within another

   d. Soiled linen is wrapped at the end of the shift

9. After taking standard precautions, a nurse starts cleaning the infected wound of a client. Which of the following sources can transmit infections diseases? Select all that apply.

   a. Blood of the infected client

   b. Sweat of the infected client

   c. Mucous membranes of the client

   d. Non-intact skin of the infected client

   e. Breath of the infected client

10. A nurse used droplet precautions for 2 weeks when caring for a client with acute rheumatic fever. The nurse knows that transmission-based precautions depend mostly on which of the following factors?

    a. The nature of the infecting microorganisms

    b. The route of transmission of the pathogen

    c. The stage of the infection in the client

    d. The treatment available for the infection

11. A nurse is cleaning the infected wound of a client, which is partially healed. When are transmission-based precautions discontinued?

    a. When culture findings are positive

    b. When a lesion stops draining

    c. When the client shows drug-resistant strains

    d. When the blood around the wound dries

12. A nurse needs to collect the urine and stool specimens of a client with acute meningococcal meningitis. Which of the following precautions should the nurse take when delivering the specimens to the laboratory?

    a. Leave some air gap in the container after collecting the specimens

    b. Wear new gloves when collecting the specimens from the client

    c. Collect and deliver the specimens in a plastic biohazard bag

    d. Collect the specimens in sealed containers and place them in a plastic biohazard bag

13. A nurse is caring for a client with tuberculosis, who is admitted to a private room in the health care facility. Which of the following infection control measures should the nurse take? Select all that apply.

    a. Close the doors and windows to control air currents

    b. Allow only one visitor at any given time to meet the client

    c. Ask housekeeping to clean the infectious client's room last

    d. Use only disposable linen and medical equipment for the infectious client

    e. Post an instruction card on the door or nearby at eye level

14. A nurse is using droplet precaution measures when caring for a client with streptococcal pharyngitis. The nurse knows that the droplet precaution will reduce pathogen transmission from the client to the nurse up to how many feet?

 a. Less than 10 feet

 b. Less than 3 feet

 c. Less than 5 feet

 d. Less than 8 feet

15. A nurse is cleaning the room of a client with open tuberculosis. The nurse has collected the soiled dressings of the client. Which of the following can be safely disposed of in landfills?

 a. Autoclaved items

 b. Unused syringes

 c. Wrapped dressings

 d. Sealed containers

16. In the health care facility, a nurse is caring for a long-term elderly client with chronic asthma and skin infections. Elderly clients are at increased risk for which of the following infectious diseases?

 a. Pneumonia

 b. Influenza

 c. Urinary tract infection

 d. AIDS

 e. Glanders

17. A nurse needs to fix a respirator mask on the face of a bearded client with tuberculosis. Which of the following respirator masks is most suitable for a bearded client?

 a. N-95 respirator

 b. Powered air-purifying respirator

 c. Ultrasonic nebulizer

 d. Nebulizer

CHAPTER 23

Body Mechanics, Positioning, and Moving

SECTION I: LEARNING OBJECTIVES

- Identify characteristics of good posture in a standing, sitting, or lying position.
- Describe three principles of correct body mechanics.
- Explain the purpose of ergonomics.
- Give at least two examples of ergonomic recommendations in the workplace.
- Describe at least 10 signs or symptoms associated with the disuse syndrome.
- Describe six common client positions.
- Explain the purpose of five different positioning devices used for safety and comfort.
- Name one advantage for each of three different pressure-relieving devices.
- Discuss four types of transfer devices.
- Give at least five general guidelines that apply to transferring clients.

SECTION II: ASSESSING YOUR UNDERSTANDING

Activity A *Fill in the blanks.*

1. The consequences of inactivity are collectively referred to as the _____ syndrome.

2. Good posture distributes _____ through the center of the body over a wide base of support.

3. Muscle _____ occur more often when muscles are strained and forced to work beyond their capacity.

4. _____ is a specialty field of engineering science devoted to promoting comfort, performance, and health in the workplace.

5. Placing a bed in a slight _____ position may help keep the client from sliding down toward the foot of the bed.

6. Bone _____ increases the risk of fractures in older adults.

7. _____ refers to moving a client from the bed to a chair, toilet, or stretcher and back to the bed again.

8. _____ are the bony protrusions at the head of the femur near the hip.

9. Foot drop hinders _____ because it interferes with a person's ability to place the heel on the floor.

Activity B *Consider the following figures.*

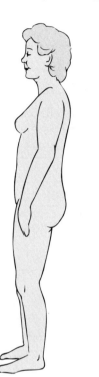

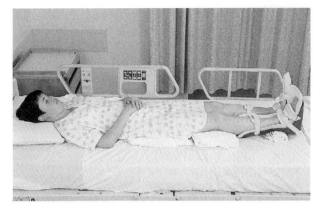

3. Identify the figure.

_____

_____

_____

4. What is this device used for?

_____

_____

_____

1. Identify the figure.

_____

_____

_____

2. What are its benefits?

_____

_____

_____

Activity C *Match the specialty beds in column A with their description in column B.*

Column A

____ **1.** Low-air loss bed

____ **2.** Air-fluidized bed

____ **3.** Oscillating support bed

____ **4.** Circular bed

Column B

A. Contains a collection of tiny beads within a mattress cover

B. The client is sandwiched between the anterior and posterior frames in a 180-degree arc

C. Contains inflated air sacs within the mattress

D. Slowly and continuously rocks the client from side to side in a 124-degree arc

Activity D *Presented here, in random order, are steps in using a transfer board to transfer a client from a bed to a chair. Write the correct sequence in the boxes provided.*

1. Angle the transfer board from the client's buttocks and hips down toward the seat of the chair.

2. Slide the client down the transfer board into the seat of the chair at an agreed-upon signal.

3. Remove an arm from the wheelchair and slide the client to the edge of the bed.

4. Support and brace the client's knee with your knees while maintaining proper body mechanics.

5. Position the transfer board beneath the client.

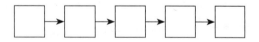

Activity E *Briefly answer the following.*

1. How is a good sitting posture maintained?

_____

_____

_____

2. What are the benefits of maintaining good body mechanics?

_____

_____

_____

3. What causes ergonomic hazards to health care workers?

_____

_____

_____

4. What are the potential problems of an air-fluidized bed?

_____

_____

_____

5. What are the effects of immobility faced by older adults?

_____

_____

_____

Activity F *Use the clues to complete the crossword puzzle.*

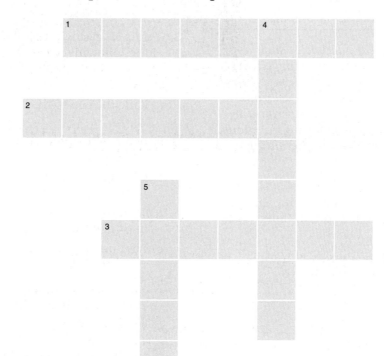

Across

1. Skeletal changes that affect the older person's center of gravity
2. Triangular piece of metal hung by a chain over the head of the bed
3. It keeps the client from sliding downward into the Trendelenburg position

Down

4. Force exerted against the surface and layers of the skin as tissues slide in opposite but parallel directions
5. This position provides good drainage from bronchioles, stretches the trunk and extremities, and keeps the hips in an extended position

SECTION III: APPLYING YOUR KNOWLEDGE

Activity G *Nursing care activities such as positioning, moving, and transferring clients reduce the potential for disuse syndrome. Nurses can become injured if they fail to use good posture and body mechanics while performing these activities. Answer the following questions, which involve the nurse's role in preventing work-related injuries.*

A nurse is caring for an elderly client with a fractured leg following a fall. When caring for this client, the nurse should take precautions to prevent injuries to him- or herself.

1. What care should the nurse take before planning to turn and move the client?

   _____

   _____

   _____

2. What should the nurse do as part of planning to move the client?

   _____

   _____

   _____

SECTION IV: PRACTICING FOR NCLEX

Activity H *Answer the following questions.*

1. A nurse is aware of the importance of maintaining a good standing posture to promote efficient use of the musculoskeletal system. Which of the following is a component of a good standing posture?
   a. Keep feet about 2 to 3 inches apart
   b. Avoid bending the knees
   c. Maintain hips at an even level
   d. Hold the chest slightly backward

2. A nurse is working at a health care facility where client data are recorded on a computer. When working at the computer terminal, which of the following are ergonomically sound actions?
   a. Use dim lights
   b. Flex elbows at 120 degrees

   c. Use a low chair
   d. Use wrist rests

3. A nurse is caring for an inactive client. Which of the following are principles of positioning that the nurse should follow? Select all that apply.
   a. Raise the bed to the height of the caregiver's elbow.
   b. Remove the pillows and positioning devices.
   c. Change the inactive client's position at least every 2 hours.
   d. Turn the upper part of the client's body and then the lower part.
   e. Lift and drag the client when transferring to a stretcher.

4. A nurse is caring for an elderly client with restricted movement. The nurse knows that placing the client in which of the following positions for long could lead to skin breakdown at the end of the spine?
   a. Prone
   b. Supine
   c. Lateral
   d. Sims'

5. A nurse is caring for a client with dyspnea. Which of the following positions allows for the exchange of a greater volume of air?
   a. Supine
   b. Sims'
   c. Fowler's
   d. Lateral

6. When caring for a client at his home, the nurse uses pillows to provide comfort and elevate a body part. Which of the following should the nurse use to elevate the upper part of the body if an adjustable bed is not available?
   a. Oversized pillows
   b. Contour pillows
   c. Triangular wedges
   d. Bolsters

7. A nurse is caring for a client who had a stroke and has restricted mobility of his right arm. Why should the nurse use hand rolls for this client?

   a. To prevent contractures of the fingers

   b. To hold the fingers in a tight fist

   c. To keep the fingers and thumb together

   d. To prevent the wrist from turning outward

8. A team of nurses is using a roller sheet to turn a client who is in the supine position to the lateral position. Which of the following should the nurses consider when using the roller sheet?

   a. Lift the client to change position

   b. Avoid stooping when turning the client

   c. Place the sheet away from the client

   d. Keep the sheet rolled on the bed after use

9. A nurse is caring for a client whose right leg has been amputated after a motor vehicle accident. With which of the following devices should the nurse provide the client to move about in bed?

   a. Foot board

   b. Bed board

   c. Trochanter roll

   d. Trapeze

10. A nurse is caring for an elderly client who has undergone surgery for cataracts. Which of the following devices is appropriate for this client's bed?

    a. Side rails

    b. Cradle

    c. Transfer handles

    d. Transfer board

11. A nurse is caring for a client who is confined to his bed at his home. The client uses a water mattress to prevent pressure ulcers. Which of the following is true for water mattresses?

    a. Distribute water cyclically

    b. Contain inflated air sacs

    c. Require a lot of time to refill

    d. Drain excretions away from the body

12. Nurses at the health care facility are required to use assistive devices whenever they are required to care for immobile clients. Which of the following is an advantage of using an assistive device for the nurse?

    a. Maintains dignity and self-esteem

    b. Reduces musculoskeletal injuries

    c. Relieves anxiety concerning safety

    d. Promotes faster recovery

13. Two nurses are using a roller sheet to move a client. Which of the following should the nurses do during the procedure?

    a. Stand on the same side of the client

    b. Lower the bed to waist level

    c. Face each other on opposite sides of the bed

    d. Place the sheet beneath the shoulders and buttocks

14. A nurse is caring for a client whose level of functional status is indicated as 4 in the health record. What does a functional status of level 4 indicate?

    a. Needs total assistance

    b. Needs total supervision

    c. Needs assistive device

    d. Needs minimal help

15. A nurse is caring for a client with severe burn injuries. The client requires frequent dressing changes and topical applications. Which of the following pressure-relieving devices should the nurse provide for this client?

    a. Oscillating support bed

    b. Foam mattress

    c. Gel cushion

    d. Circular bed

CHAPTER 24

Therapeutic Exercise

SECTION I: LEARNING OBJECTIVES

- List at least five benefits of regular exercise.
- Define fitness.
- Identify seven factors that interfere with fitness.
- Name at least two methods of fitness testing.
- Describe how to calculate a person's target heart rate.
- Define metabolic energy equivalent.
- Differentiate fitness exercise from therapeutic exercise.
- Differentiate isotonic exercise from isometric exercise.
- Give at least one example of isotonic and isometric exercises.
- Differentiate between active exercise and passive exercise.
- Discuss how and why range-of-motion (ROM) exercises are performed.
- Provide at least two suggestions for helping older adults become or stay physically active.

SECTION II: ASSESSING YOUR UNDERSTANDING

Activity A *Fill in the blanks.*

1. _____ or purposeful physical activity is beneficial to people of all age groups.

2. Body _____ is the amount of body tissue that is lean versus the amount that is fat.

3. The validity of _____ tests is less reliable than results obtained through ECG testing.

4. _____ heart rate means the goal for heart rate during exercise.

5. _____ energy equivalent is the measure of energy and oxygen consumption during exercise.

6. _____ exercise involves rhythmically moving all parts of the body at a moderate to slow speed without hindering the ability to breathe.

7. _____ exercise is therapeutic activity that the client performs independently after proper instruction.

Activity B *Consider the following figures.*

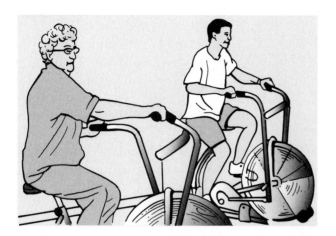

1. Identify the figure.

_____

_____

_____

2. What is the benefit of this type of activity?

_____

_____

_____

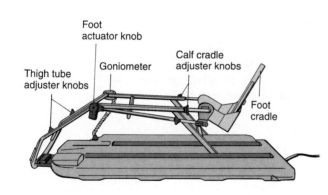

3. Identify the figure.

_____

_____

_____

4. What is this device used for?

_____

_____

_____

Activity C *Match the positions in column A with the descriptions in column B.*

Column A

____ **1.** Hyperex-
tension

____ **2.** Abduction

____ **3.** Rotation

____ **4.** Pronation

____ **5.** Inversion

Column B

A. Turning downward

B. Increasing the angle between two adjoining bones more than 180 degrees

C. Turning the sole of the foot toward the midline

D. Turning from side to side, as in an arc

E. Moving away from the midline

Activity D *Briefly answer the following.*

1. What are the factors that can affect a client's fitness and stamina?

_____

_____

_____

2. Why are fitness tests important?

_____

_____

_____

3. What is recovery index?

_____

_____

_____

4. How is a walk-a-mile test conducted?

_____

_____

_____

5. How is the maximum heart rate calculated?

_____

_____

_____

Activity E *Use the clues to complete the crossword puzzle.*

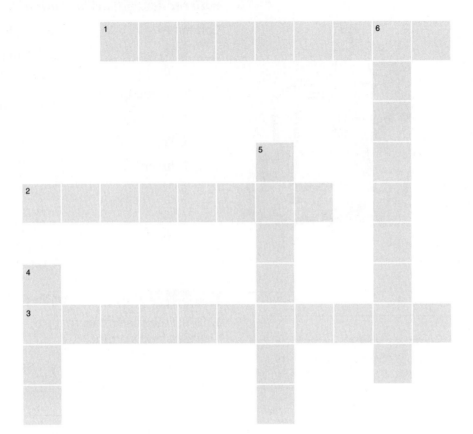

Across

1. Permanent loss of joint movement
2. Type of exercise involving movement and work
3. Exercises performed by people with health risks

Down

4. A submaximal fitness test
5. The capacity to exercise
6. Stationary exercises generally performed against a resistive force

SECTION III: APPLYING YOUR KNOWLEDGE

Activity F *Nurses are responsible for assessing each client's fitness level before initiating an exercise program with the client. Exercise must be individualized per the need and fitness ability of the client. Answer the following questions, which involve the nurse's role in assisting the client in a safe exercise program.*

1. What are the initial requirements of which the nurse should inform the client before starting an exercise program?

   _____

   _____

   _____

2. What kind of activities should the nurse suggest for a client with a metabolic energy equivalent to 6 to 7 METs?

   _____

   _____

SECTION IV: PRACTICING FOR NCLEX

Activity G *Answer the following questions.*

1. A nurse is assisting an immobile client to perform ROM exercises. Which of the following should the nurse keep in mind when performing ROM exercises? Select all that apply.
   a. Raise the level of the bed
   b. Repeat each exercise five times
   c. Avoid forceful joint movements
   d. Begin with foot exercises and work upward
   e. Move the client closer to the edge of the bed

2. A nurse is caring for a client who has been prescribed isometric exercises. Which of the following is a benefit of isometric exercises?
   a. Preserving muscle mass
   b. Preventing joint deformities
   c. Preventing stiffness of joints
   d. Preventing skin breakdown

3. A client has been recommended isotonic exercises by the health care provider. Which of the following exercises is an isotonic exercise?
   a. Body building
   b. Weight lifting
   c. Stationary cycling
   d. Aerobics

4. A nurse is caring for a client who has undergone a mastectomy. Which of the following exercises should the nurse recommend to the client to strengthen the arm on the surgical side? Select all that apply.
   a. Squeezing a softball
   b. Combing the hair
   c. Swimming
   d. Finger climbing
   e. Rotating the arm

5. Before starting the client on a suitable exercise routine, the nurse is required to assess the client's fitness. Which of the following assessment techniques will provide reliable results for fitness levels?
   a. Walk-a-mile test
   b. Step test
   c. ECG
   d. Aerobic fitness

6. A nurse is caring for an elderly client with diabetes who has been asked to exercise on a regular basis. Which of the following exercises would be ideal for this client?
   a. Walking
   b. Cycling
   c. Running
   d. Jogging

7. When preparing an exercise regimen for an elderly client and instructing the client on a safe exercise program, which of the following should the nurse tell the client?
   a. Avoid drinking water just before exercising
   b. Take sips of aerated drinks during the exercise program
   c. Balance periods of physical activity with periods of rest
   d. Wear shoes with a smooth sole for easy walking

8. A nurse is assessing a client for unilateral neglect. Which of the following would confirm unilateral neglect in the client?

   a. The client constantly ignores objects placed on his left side

   b. The client differentiates warm and cold on both sides

   c. The client combs his hair well on both sides

   d. The client observes objects on the table on either side

9. A client who has undergone knee replacement therapy has been ordered the use of a passive motion machine as a substitute for manual ROM exercise. What care should the nurse take when caring for this client? Select all that apply.

   a. Provide pain medication after exercise is completed

   b. Instruct the client on techniques for relaxation

   c. Compare assessment findings with the unaffected extremity

   d. Assess vital signs and mobility of the affected extremity

   e. Adjust the machine to the prescribed rate and degree of flexion

10. When caring for a client with unilateral neglect, the client is always aware of activities on the right hand side. Which of the following interventions should the nurse follow?

    a. Suggest that the client view the environment from one side

    b. Place the signal cord on the left side of the client

    c. Avoid asking the client to participate in self-care for the left side

    d. Always approach the client from the right side

11. A nurse is assisting a client in performing ROM exercises. The nurse assists the client to move the arm in a full circle. With which of the following exercises is the nurse assisting the client?

    a. Flexion

    b. Extension

    c. Circumduction

    d. Hyperextension

12. A client is to undergo an ambulatory ECG to record heart rate and rhythm continuously during normal activity. Which of the following should the nurse tell the client?

    a. Wear the Holter monitor for 12 hours

    b. Walk slowly first on a flat treadmill

    c. Measure peripheral oxygenation

    d. Avoid the use of electric blankets

13. A client has been ordered a step test, which is a submaximal fitness test involving a timed stepping activity. Which of the following is true for this test?

    a. The platform height is 30 inches for men

    b. The platform height is 16 inches for men

    c. A step up and down together is one step

    d. The exercise involves about 76 steps per minute

14. A nurse is caring for a client whose cardiovascular endurance fitness level is 60. How should the nurse classify this fitness level?

    a. Poor

    b. Below average

    c. Average

    d. Good

15. A nurse is assisting a client to perform ROM exercises. Which of the following should the nurse do when assisting the client?

    a. Provide the client with pillows

    b. Move each joint until there is pain

    c. Support the joint being exercised

    d. Follow a different pattern each time

Mechanical Immobilization

SECTION I: LEARNING OBJECTIVES

- List at least three purposes of mechanical immobilization.
- Name four types of splints.
- Discuss why slings and braces are used.
- Explain the purpose of a cast.
- Name three types of casts.
- Describe at least five nursing actions that are appropriate when caring for clients with casts.
- Discuss how casts are removed.
- Explain what traction implies.
- List three types of traction.
- Name seven principles that apply to maintaining effective traction.
- Describe the purpose for an external fixator.
- Identify the rationale for performing pin site care.

SECTION II: ASSESSING YOUR UNDERSTANDING

Activity A *Fill in the blanks.*

1. A(n) _____ cast encircles one or both arms or legs and the chest or the trunk.

2. A(n) _____ is a cloth device used to elevate, cradle, and support parts of the body.

3. _____ are custom-made or custom-fitted devices designed to support weakened structures such as weak muscles or unstable joints.

4. A(n) _____ cast encircles an arm or leg and leaves the toes or fingers exposed.

5. _____ is a pulling effect exerted on a part of the skeletal system.

6. An external _____ is a metal device inserted into and through one or more broken bones to stabilize fragments.

7. _____ fractures are common, especially in post-menopausal women who are not treated for osteoporosis.

8. _____ traction is most often used briefly to realign a broken bone.

9. The pull of the traction generally is offset by the _____ from the client's own body weight.

10. A light-cured _____ cast requires exposure to ultraviolet light to harden.

Activity B *Consider the following figures.*

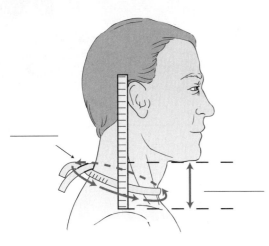

1. Identify and label the image.

   _____

   _____

   _____

2. What is this procedure used for?

   _____

   _____

   _____

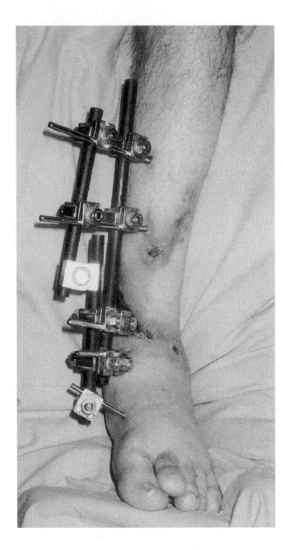

3. Identify the image.

   _____

   _____

   _____

4. What is the use of the metal device in this procedure?

   _____

   _____

   _____

Activity C *Match the mechanical immobilization devices in column A with their features in column B.*

Column A

____ **1.** Thomas splint

____ **2.** Makeshift splint

____ **3.** Pelvic belt

____ **4.** Ice pack

Column B

A. Applied to the lower extremity

B. Pulling effect on the skeletal system

C. Applied to alleviate pain

D. Board, broom, handle, or golf club

Activity D *Presented here, in random order, are steps that occur when applying an arm sling. Write the correct sequence in the boxes provided.*

1. Position the forearm across the client's chest with the thumb upward.

2. Slip the flexed arm into the canvas sling so that the elbow fits flush.

3. Tighten the strap to keep the elbow flexed and the wrist elevated.

4. Assess the skin color and temperature of the injured arm.

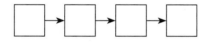

Activity E *Briefly answer the following.*

1. What are the disadvantages of plaster of paris casts?

_____

_____

_____

2. What is the purpose of mechanical immobilization?

_____

_____

_____

3. What is the function of splints?

_____

_____

_____

4. What are the dangers of indwelling catheters in older adults?

_____

_____

_____

5. Why is care at the pin site essential?

_____

_____

_____

6. What skin care needs to be taken after removing a cast?

_____

_____

_____

Activity F *Use the clues to complete the crossword puzzle.*

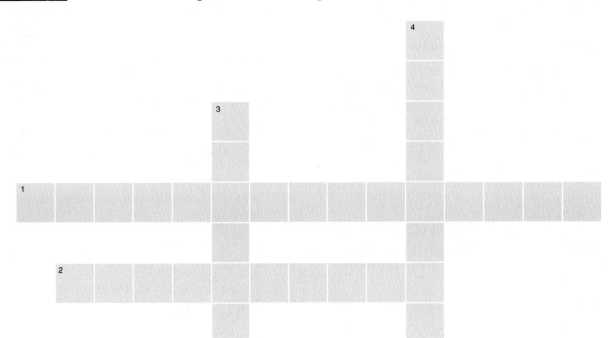

Across

1. These injuries are painful and heal slowly compared with the skin or soft tissue
2. Cast edges that may be sharp and cause skin abrasions

Down

3. Straps made of this material are used to secure cervical collars
4. This injury has reduced because of the use of neck supports in automobiles

SECTION III: APPLYING YOUR KNOWLEDGE

Activity G *External fixators are inserted into and through one or more broken bones to stabilize fragments during healing. Although the external fixator immobilizes the area of injury, the client is encouraged to be active and mobile. During recovery, the nurse provides care for the pin sites. In conjunction with an external fixator and skeletal traction, pin site care is essential to prevent infection. Answer the following questions, which involve the nurse's role in caring for a client with an external fixator.*

A nurse is taking care of a client with pin sites. A culture from a specimen taken at a pin site reveals that the pin site is infected with *Staphylococcus aureus*.

1. What nursing actions are required for contact precautions to control transmission of the pathogen?

   _____

   _____

   _____

2. How should the nurse assess a client with pin site insertion in his or her body?

   _____

   _____

   _____

SECTION IV: PRACTICING FOR NCLEX

Activity H *Answer the following questions.*

1. A nurse has finished applying a cast to a client. Which of the following actions should the nurse perform to reduce the pain and swelling?
   a. Elevate the cast on pillows or other supports
   b. Administer pain relief medication
   c. Provide written instructions on cast care
   d. Place the bed at a comfortable height

2. A nurse is caring for a client with injury to his right leg. Which of the following is most suitable for short-term duration? Select all that apply.
   a. Pneumatic splints
   b. Immobilizers
   c. Thomas splints
   d. Molded splints
   e. Russell's traction

3. A nurse is assessing a client with a pin inserted in a fractured femur. The client's pin insertion site shows no evidence of purulent drainage. What other signs should the nurse look for to check for pin site infection?
   a. Check whether the pin is bent
   b. Check white blood cell count
   c. Check for dry skin
   d. Check the client's pulse rate

4. A nurse has applied a molded splint to the sprained ankle of a client. What will be the desired outcome of applying a molded splint? Select all that apply.
   a. Reduce the load-bearing force on the cervical spine
   b. Maintain the body part in a functional position
   c. Prevent contractures and muscle atrophy during immobility
   d. Immobilize the injured structure and align it

5. A nurse is trimming a cast in the anal and genital area so that the client can eliminate urine and stool. Which of the following casts is the nurse trimming?
   a. Cylinder cast
   b. Spica cast
   c. Bivalved cast
   d. Body cast

6. A nurse is caring for an elderly client with musculoskeletal injury near the hip. Which of the following should the nurse do to promote the quick healing of a musculoskeletal injury?
   a. Encourage the client to have a diet rich in protein, calcium, and zinc
   b. Encourage the client to protect himself or herself from exposure to sun
   c. Ask the client to avoid taking supplements of vitamin D
   d. Encourage the client to perform isometric exercise daily

7. A nurse has removed the cast applied to the forearm of a client. Which of the following physical changes should the affected area show after removal of the cast?
   a. Joints have better flexibility
   b. Skin appears pale and waxy
   c. Unexercised muscles appear bigger
   d. Major swelling appears on the affected area

8. A nurse needs to apply Buck's traction to a client with severe muscle spasms in his leg. Which of the following actions is performed when applying Buck's traction to a client?
   a. A pulling effect caused by the use of the hands and muscular strength
   b. A pulling effect caused on the skeletal system by devices
   c. A pulling exerted directly by devices through bone
   d. A pulling effect caused by a metal device inserted into broken bone

9. A nurse is caring for an elderly client with a fractured hip. Which of the following reasons explains why hip fractures are common in the elderly?
   a. Weakness of bone
   b. Poor diet
   c. Reduced synovial fluid
   d. Flexible joints

10. A nurse is applying a custom-made leg brace to the client. What will happen if the brace is ill-fitting or applied improperly? Select all that apply.

    a. Causes discomfort

    b. Causes skin ulcerations

    c. Causes deformity

    d. Causes permanent stiffness

    e. Causes muscle contractures

11. A client whose neck has been in traction for 10 minutes tells the nurse that he feels tired and exhausted. The nurse knows that which of the following is best for the client?

    a. Avoid giving a pillow to the client

    b. Reduce the amount of weights

    c. Use a pressure-relieving device

    d. Change the position of the client

12. A nurse is caring for a client who has an injured elbow. Which of the following nursing actions should the nurse remember to facilitate circulation?

    a. Slip the flexed arm in the canvas sling

    b. Avoid more than 90 degrees of flexion

    c. Position the triangle apex under the elbow

    d. Position the knot near the neck side

13. Per the physician's orders, a nurse is prematurely removing the cast of a client with a fractured arm. Under what circumstances does the nurse know it is appropriate to remove a cast prematurely:

    a. When complications develop

    b. When the injury is healed sufficiently

    c. When the cast edges become soft

    d. When there is a need for hygiene

14. A nurse is assisting a client with a hip spica cast during elimination. The nurse knows that which of the following actions will protect the spica cast from soiling?

    a. Tuck in an adult diaper

    b. Provide a bedpan

    c. Insert a catheter

    d. Use plastic wrap

15. A nurse is assisting a physician in applying a pneumatic splint to the severely injured leg of a client. How should the nurse know the point up to which the pneumatic splint needs to be inflated with air?

    a. Ask the client if the splint feels heavy

    b. Touch the splint and determine whether it is cold

    c. Determine whether the splint can be indented a half inch

    d. Push a fingertip between the splint and leg

16. A nurse is administering prescribed medicine to an elderly client with a fractured hip. Which of the following effects of narcotic analgesics will be visible in elderly adults? Select all that apply.

    a. Pale skin

    b. Dilated pupils

    c. Constipation

    d. Depressed respiration

    e. Mental changes

17. A client accidentally pours a glassful of water on the cast. The nurse quickly dries the cast using a blow dryer set on a cool setting. Which other types of basic care should the nurse provide when caring for a client with a cast?

    a. Keep clients from writing anything on the cast

    b. Avoid elevating the cast on a pillow or support

    c. Apply heat packs to the cast at the level of injury

    d. Avoid ambulating clients until the injury is healed

18. A nurse is caring for a client who is in Russell's traction for long-term treatment. Which of the following actions should the nurse perform to maintain the client's personal hygiene?

    a. Clean the skin around insertion site

    b. Cover the metal pins with corks

    c. Bathe the back of the client

    d. Insert padding within the slings

Ambulatory Aids

SECTION I: LEARNING OBJECTIVES

- Name four activities that prepare clients for ambulation.
- Give two examples of isometric exercises that tone and strengthen the lower extremities.
- Identify one technique for building upper arm strength.
- Explain the reason for dangling clients or using a tilt table.
- Name two devices used to assist clients with ambulation.
- Give three examples of ambulatory aids.
- Identify the most stable type of ambulatory aid.
- Describe three characteristics of appropriately fitted crutches.
- Name four types of crutch-walking gaits.
- Explain the purpose of a temporary prosthetic limb.
- Discuss two criteria that must be met before constructing a permanent prosthetic limb.
- Name four components of above-the-knee and below-the-knee prosthetic limbs.
- Describe how a prosthetic limb is applied.
- Discuss age-related changes that affect the gait and ambulation of older adults.

SECTION II: ASSESSING YOUR UNDERSTANDING

Activity A *Fill in the blanks.*

1. _____ exercises are used to promote muscle tone and strength.

2. _____ helps to normalize blood pressure, which may drop when the client rises from a reclining position.

3. A client who has weakness on one side of the body uses a(n) _____, which is a hand-held ambulatory device made of wood or aluminum.

4. _____ crutches are generally used by experienced clients who need permanent assistance with walking.

5. Many clients with _____ use platform crutches.

6. The word *point* in four-point gait refers to the _____ of the crutches and legs used when performing a gait.

7. Clients with leg amputation ambulate with a _____ limb without the assistance of crutches or other ambulatory aids.

8. _____ crutches are used by clients who cannot bear weight with their hands and wrists.

9. The use of assistive devices for mobility may cause _____ in older adults.

10. Clients who need temporary assistance with ambulation are likely to use _____ crutches.

Activity B *Consider the following figure.*

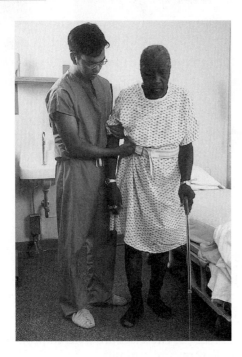

1. Identify the assistive device used to help the client ambulate.

_____

_____

_____

2. How does a nurse assist the client ambulate using this assistive device?

_____

_____

_____

Activity C *Match the terms to ambulatory aids in column A with their description in column B.*

Column A

____ 1. Quadriceps setting

____ 2. Parallel bars

____ 3. T-handle cane

____ 4. Forearm crutches

Column B

A. Used as hand rails to gain practice in ambulating

B. Have an arm cuff but do not have an axillary bar

C. An isometric exercise during which the client alternately tenses and relaxes the quadriceps muscles

D. Has a handgrip with a slightly bent shaft, offering users more stability

Activity D *Presented here, in random order, are the instructions a nurse gives to a client who uses a walker. Write the correct sequence in the boxes provided.*

1. Take a step forward.

2. Support the body weight on the handgrips when moving the weaker leg.

3. Hold on to the walker at the padded handgrips.

4. Stand within the walker.

5. Pick up the walker and advance it 6 to 8 inches (15–20 cm)

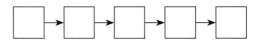

Activity E *Briefly answer the following.*

1. What are the techniques that a nurse can use to increase muscular strength and the ability to bear weight?

_____

_____

_____

2. What is the function of the quadriceps muscles?

_____

_____

3. What does an exercise regimen to strengthen the upper arm include?

_____

_____

_____

4. What is a tilt table?

_____

_____

_____

5. How is the correct height of the cane for a client achieved?

_____

_____

_____

6. What is the importance of the immediate post-operative prosthesis?

_____

_____

_____

Activity F *Use the clues to complete the crossword puzzle.*

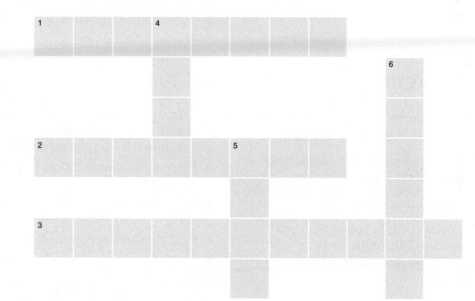

Across

1. An ambulatory aid constructed of wood or aluminum generally used in pairs
2. The power to perform
3. The condition of clients who require physical conditioning before they ambulate again

Down

4. The ability of the muscles to respond when stimulated
5. Manner of walking
6. Used by a client who requires considerable support and assistance with balance

SECTION III: APPLYING YOUR KNOWLEDGE

Activity G *A prosthetic limb allows clients with leg amputation to ambulate without the assistance of crutches or other ambulatory aids. Answer the questions related to nursing intervention for a client with prosthetic limbs.*

A nurse is caring for a client whose right leg was amputated as a result of gangrene. The client has been fitted with a temporary prosthetic limb immediately after the surgery.

1. What procedure should the nurse apply when fitting a client with a prosthetic limb?

   _____

   _____

   _____

2. What are the responsibilities of the nurse to ensure that no complications develop?

   _____

   _____

   _____

SECTION IV: PRACTICING FOR NCLEX

Activity H *Answer the following questions.*

1. A nurse is caring for a client who temporarily lost the function of his legs as a result of a motor vehicle accident. How can the nurse prepare the client for ambulation?

   a. By assisting the client in performing isometric exercises of the upper arms

   b. By assisting the client in walking using a supportive belt

   c. By using a tilt table to help the client stand

   d. By assisting the client in performing isotonic exercises of the lower limbs

2. A nurse needs to prepare a client for ambulation whose leg is in a cast as a result of a hairline fracture. Which of the following would

help the client to re-establish her previous ability to walk?

   a. Walking belts

   b. Isometric exercises

   c. Dangling

   d. Tilt table

3. A nurse is assisting a middle-age client who has been admitted to the facility with diarrhea. The client is weak and in the recovery stage. Why should the nurse assist the client to dangle before ambulating?

   a. To promote muscle tone and strength

   b. To improve upper arm strength

   c. To normalize the blood pressure

   d. To help the client bear weight on his or her feet

4. A nurse is caring for a client who is being treated at the health care facility for a torn muscle fiber in the quadriceps. The nurse should understand that which of the following is the function of the quadriceps?

   a. Aids in supporting body weight

   b. Aids in adducting the leg

   c. Aids in rotating the leg

   d. Aids in walking upright

5. A client is being treated for injury to the gluteal muscle. The physician has prescribed exercises in a gluteal setting to rehabilitate the client. How should the client exercise the gluteal muscles in a gluteal setting?

   a. By practicing ambulation with the help of hand rails

   b. By performing modified hand pushups in bed

   c. By sitting on the edge of the bed

   d. By contracting and relaxing the muscles

6. A client has been prescribed modified hand pushups in bed to strengthen the upper arms because she will have to use axillary crutches for a while after discharge from the facility. What should the nurse do if the mattress of the bed is soft?

   a. Remove the mattress from the bed

   b. Replace the mattress with a firmer one

   c. Place books under the client's hand

   d. Provide the client with a sturdy arm chair

7. When applying a prosthetic limb to a client at the health care facility, what instruction should the nurse give to the client to prevent circulatory problems?
   a. Ask the client to wear a nylon sheath beneath the stump sock
   b. Ask the client to avoid keeping the knee naturally flexed for a prolonged period
   c. Ask the client to dry the socks well before donning them
   d. Ask the client to wear the prosthesis for a short period initially

8. When using a tilt table to prepare a client for ambulation, when is the table lowered and returned to the horizontal position?
   a. When the client appears to be dizzy
   b. When the table has been tilted to 30 degrees
   c. When the client is in a vertical position
   d. When the device has been used for more than 10 minutes

9. When ambulating the client, the nurse notices that the client appears dizzy and is about to faint. What should the nurse do in this case? Select all that apply.
   a. Slide an arm under the client's axilla
   b. Balance the client on his or her hip
   c. Slide the client down to the floor
   d. Place the client on the bed
   e. Go and fetch water for the client

10. A nurse at the health care facility is caring for clients who are beginning to ambulate and may require the help of an ambulatory aid. In which of the following cases could a nurse suggest the use of a cane to a client to aid ambulation?
    a. Clients who have weakness on one side of the body
    b. Clients who require considerable assistance with balance
    c. Clients who need brief, temporary assistance ambulating
    d. Clients who need permanent assistance when walking

11. A nurse is caring for a client who has a fractured leg in a cast. Which of the following ambulatory devices could the nurse use to aid this client to ambulate?
    a. Cane
    b. Axillary crutch

c. Walker
d. Platform crutch

12. A nurse is caring for a client whose legs have been amputated from below the knee. Which of the following components form part of the below-the-knee-prosthesis? Select all that apply.
    a. Socket
    b. Shank
    c. Ankle/foot system
    d. Knee system
    e. Lightweight tube

13. Listed here, in random order, are the steps followed when a client with a walker has to sit down in an armchair. Arrange the steps in the proper order.
    a. Release the grip of the walker
    b. Grip the armrest of the chair
    c. Lower himself or herself in the chair
    d. Grasp the opposite armrest

14. Listed here, in random order, are the steps followed when a client with a walker has to get up from the armchair. Arrange the steps in the proper order.
    a. Reposition the walker
    b. Push up on the armrest with both arms
    c. Move to the edge of the chair
    d. Use one hand to grasp the walker and place the other on the armrest

15. Which of the following clients who use crutches to ambulate would have a swing-through gait?
    a. A paralyzed client with leg braces
    b. An amputee learning to use prosthesis
    c. A client with a severe ankle sprain
    d. A client who has more strength and balance

16. An arthritic client who uses crutches to ambulate is being treated at the health care facility. Which of the following gaits would the nurse observe when this client ambulates using the crutches?
    a. Four-point
    b. Two-point
    c. Three-point non-weight bearing
    d. Three-point partial-weight bearing

CHAPTER 27

Perioperative Care

SECTION I: LEARNING OBJECTIVES

- Define perioperative care.
- Identify the three phases of perioperative care.
- Differentiate inpatient from outpatient surgery.
- List at least four advantages of laser surgery.
- Discuss two methods for donating blood before surgery.
- Identify four major activities that nurses perform for all clients immediately before surgery.
- Name three topics to address during preoperative teaching.
- Explain the purpose of antiembolism stockings.
- Name three methods for removing hair when preparing the skin for surgery.
- List at least five items that are verified on the preoperative checklist.
- Name three parts of the surgical department used during the intraoperative period.
- Describe the focus of nursing care during the immediate post-operative period.
- Give four examples of common post-operative complications.
- Discuss the purpose of a pneumatic compression device.
- Describe at least two items of information included in discharge instructions for post-surgical clients.
- Discuss at least two ways in which the surgical care of older adults differs from that of other age groups.

SECTION II: ASSESSING YOUR UNDERSTANDING

Activity A *Fill in the blanks.*

1. _____ surgery is the term used for procedures performed on a client who is expected to stay at the facility at least overnight.

2. _____ surgery is the term used for operative procedures performed on clients who return home the same day.

3. Receiving one's own blood is called a(n) _____ transfusion.

4. _____ technology requires unique safety precautions such as eye, fire, heat, and vapor protection.

5. Shaving causes tiny cuts, also known as _____, that provide an entrance for microorganisms.

6. A(n) _____ bladder increases the risks of bladder trauma and may cause difficulty in performing the procedure of inserting an indwelling urinary catheter.

7. When a laser is used, it releases _____, which may contain intact cells.

8. _____ preparation should begin as soon as the client is aware that surgery is necessary.

9. A(n) _____ checklist identifies the status of essential presurgical activities and is completed before surgery.

10. _____ drugs are medications that counteract the effects of those used for conscious sedation.

Activity B *Consider the following figure.*

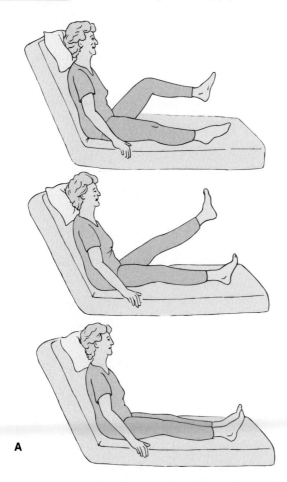

A

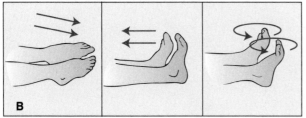

B

1. Identify the image.

_____

_____

_____

2. What are the benefits of the different positions shown in the figure?

_____

_____

_____

Activity C *Match the types of anesthesia in column A with their description in column B.*

Column A

____ **1.** General

____ **2.** Regional

____ **3.** Local

____ **4.** Topical

____ **5.** Spinal

Column B

A. Blocks sensation in a particular area without affecting consciousness

B. Inhibits sensation in skin and mucous membranes where applied directly

C. Eliminates sensation in the lower extremities, lower abdomen, and pelvis

D. Blocks sensation in a circumscribed area of skin and subcutaneous tissue

E. Eliminates all sensation and consciousness of or memory of an event

Activity D *Presented here, in random order, are the steps that occur during initial postoperative assessments. Write the correct sequence in the boxes provided.*

1. Vital signs

2. Condition of wound and dressing

3. Level of consciousness

4. Effectiveness of respirations

5. Presence of urinary catheter and urine volume

6. Location of pain and need for analgesia

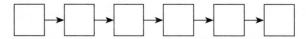

Activity E *Briefly answer the following.*

1. Why should a nurse assess a client's support system before discharge?

_____

_____

_____

2. What should a nurse do for effective wound management?

_____

_____

_____

3. When does a preoperative period start and end?

_____

_____

4. What is plume?

_____

_____

_____

5. How is consent obtained if a client is under the influence of drugs?

_____

_____

_____

6. What procedure should nurses follow regarding valuables?

_____

_____

_____

Activity F *Use the clues to complete the crossword puzzle.*

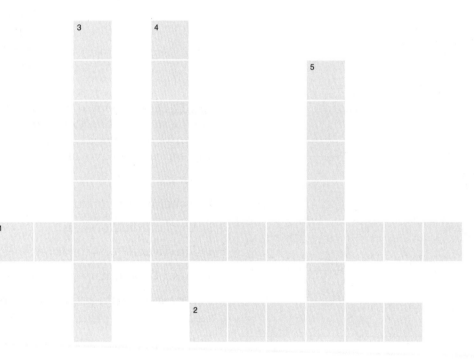

Across

1. A type of stocking used to prevent thrombi and emboli
2. A sedative promoting sleep or conscious sedation

Down

3. It keeps the bladder empty during surgery
4. An antibiotic that destroys enteric micro-organisms
5. Safety equipment worn by all during laser surgery

SECTION III: APPLYING YOUR KNOWLEDGE

Activity G *Nurses need to insert an indwelling urinary catheter preoperatively for some surgeries, particularly of the lower abdomen. If a catheter is not inserted, the nurse instructs the client to urinate immediately before receiving preoperative medication. Answer the following questions, which involve the nurse's role in preoperative care.*

A nurse is caring for a client who is scheduled for pelvic surgery. The client has undertaken skin care by cleaning the affected area with soap for several days before surgery.

1. How can the nurse ensure that the client has a clean bowel before the surgery?

   _____

   _____

   _____

2. Why is a clean bowel important during surgery?

   _____

   _____

   _____

SECTION IV: PRACTICING FOR NCLEX

Activity H *Answer the following questions.*

1. A nurse is assessing a client with a superficial cyst near the ear. Removal of the cyst can be classified as which of the following types of surgery?
   a. Optional
   b. Elective
   c. Urgent
   d. Emergency

2. A nurse is assisting a physician during a breast biopsy. For which of the following purposes is a biopsy performed?
   a. For the improvement of appearance or correction of defects
   b. For the removal of defective tissue to restore function
   c. For the enhancement of function without cure
   d. For the removal and study of tissue to make a diagnosis

3. A nurse is preparing the discharge sheet of an outpatient client. When is an outpatient client discharged? Select all that apply.
   a. When the client is awake and alert
   b. When the client is out of anesthesia
   c. When the client's oral fluids are retained
   d. When the client is able to walk independently
   e. When the client's vital signs are stable

4. A nurse is applying antiembolism stockings to a client who will undergo surgery for venous stasis ulcers. Which of the following actions should the nurse perform?
   a. Massage the legs before applying the stockings
   b. Remove the stockings once during the day and then reapply
   c. Lower the legs before applying the stockings
   d. Turn the stockings inside out before applying

5. A directed blood donor has come to the health care facility to donate blood. The nurse knows that which of the following criteria is applicable for directed blood donation?
   a. The donor should be at least 17 years of age
   b. The donor should have a hematocrit level within a safe range
   c. The donor should donate 3 to 40 days before date of use
   d. The donor should have received a blood transfusion within the past 6 months

6. A nurse is preparing a client to perform forced coughing. Which of the following clients are most appropriate for trying the forced coughing technique? Select all that apply.
   a. Clients who have moist lung sounds
   b. Clients who raise thick sputum
   c. Clients with chronic back pain
   d. Clients with abdominal incisions
   e. Clients with severe muscle spasms

7. A nurse is completing the preoperative check-list of a client scheduled for a cholecystec-tomy. What is the main purpose of a preoperative checklist before a surgery?

   a. It identifies the status of essential presurgi-cal activities.

   b. It identifies the type of surgery required for the client.

   c. It prepares the client spiritually, emotion-ally, and physically.

   d. It allows the nurse to monitor the client for complications.

8. A nurse is caring for a client during the intra-operative period. Which of the following activities are done during the intraoperative period?

   a. Transporting the client to a receiving room then on to the operating room

   b. Determining whether the client has devel-oped any allergies

   c. Preparing the client psychosocially before surgery

   d. Checking for the completion of skin preparation

9. The abdominal surgery of a client has been delayed because of an incomplete preopera-tive checklist submitted by a nurse. Which of the following could be responsible for an incomplete preoperative checklist?

   a. Unavailability of surgical equipment

   b. Improper documentation of physical examination

   c. Agency policy and availability of anesthesi-ologist

   d. Unavailability of well-fitting dentures for the client

10. A nurse is assisting a physician who is per-forming laser surgery on a client with cata-racts. Laser surgery can be used as an alternative to which other conventional surgical techniques? Select all that apply.

   a. Reattaching the retina

   b. Revascularizing ischemic heart muscle

   c. Replacing decayed teeth

   d. Removing skin tattoos

   e. Replacing and adjusting dislocated bones

11. A physician has ordered a nurse to administer regional anesthesia to a client to clean his severely infected leg injury. Which of the fol-lowing are advantages of regional anesthesia?

   a. Promotes relaxation without any sedative

   b. Avoids continuous monitoring

   c. Increases mobility of anesthetized area

   d. Decreases the risk of respiratory complication

12. A nurse is caring for a client who has devel-oped a post-operative complication of airway occlusion. Which of the following interven-tions should the nurse perform for this client?

   a. Administer prescribed intravenous fluid

   b. Place the client in the Trendelenburg position

   c. Tilt the client's head and lift the chin

   d. Insert a nasogastric tube very gently

13. A nurse is applying a pneumatic compression device to a client with impaired circulation in his lower extremity. Which of the following actions should the nurse perform?

   a. Help the client into a lateral position

   b. Palpate the pedal pulses

   c. Secure the air pump above the bed

   d. Stack and compress the air tubes

14. A nurse is writing discharge instructions for a client who has undergone exploratory laparos-copy. Which of the following factors should be addressed in the discharge instructions?

   a. How to identify purulent drainage

   b. How to assess level of pain

   c. How to care for the incision site

   d. How to ensure a patent airway

15. A nurse has to administer prescribed preop-erative medications to a client. Which of the following precautions should the nurse take before administering prescribed preoperative medications to a client? Select all that apply.

   a. Check the client's ID bracelet

   b. Allay the client's fears about the surgery

   c. Explain the process of surgery

   d. Obtain and record vital signs

   e. Ask about allergies, if any

16. A nurse is assessing the condition of an elderly client before surgery. Which of the following considerations should the nurse address as a preoperative consideration for the elderly client?

    a. Can be prone to allergies

    b. Can be susceptible to urinary tract infection

    c. May be on anticoagulation therapy

    d. May have impaired circulation and oxygenation

17. A nurse is assisting a physician during laser surgery. Which of the following precautions should the nurse take? Select all that apply.

    a. Use alcohol and acetone during surgery

    b. Ensure that black-coated surgical instruments are used

    c. Ensure that the client's teeth are covered with plastic

    d. Remove all the jewelry and metal from body

    e. Avoid using prescription glasses with shields

18. A nurse needs to perform presurgical skin preparation on a middle-age client for rectal surgery. Which of the following actions should the nurse perform as part of presurgical skin preparation?

    a. Apply moisturizer to the skin

    b. Use electric hair clippers

    c. Use a depilatory agent

    d. Assess the condition of the hair

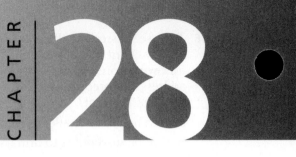

Wound Care

SECTION I: LEARNING OBJECTIVES

- Define the term *wound*.
- Name three phases of wound repair.
- Identify five signs and symptoms classically associated with the inflammatory response.
- Discuss the purpose of phagocytosis, including the two types of cells involved.
- Name three ways in which the integrity of a wound is restored.
- Explain first-, second-, and third-intention healing.
- Name two types of wounds.
- State at least three purposes for using a dressing.
- Explain the rationale for keeping wounds moist.
- Describe two types of drains, including the purpose of each.
- Name the two major methods for securing surgical wounds together until they heal.
- Explain three reasons for using a bandage or binder.
- Discuss the purpose for using one type of binder.
- Give examples of four methods used to remove non-living tissue from a wound.
- List three commonly irrigated structures.
- State two uses each for applying heat and for applying cold.
- Identify at least four methods for applying heat and cold.
- List at least five risk factors for developing pressure ulcers.
- Discuss three techniques for preventing pressure ulcers.

SECTION II: ASSESSING YOUR UNDERSTANDING

Activity A *Fill in the blanks.*

1. A(n) _____ is damaged skin or soft tissue that results from trauma.

2. _____ is the physiologic defense immediately after tissue injury that lasts for approximately 2 to 5 days.

3. _____ is a process by which the white blood cells consume pathogens, coagulated blood, and cellular debris.

4. _____ is the period during which new cells fill and seal a wound, and it occurs from 2 days to 3 weeks after the inflammatory phase.

5. _____ follows the proliferative phase and may last 6 months to 2 years.

6. _____ debridement is appropriate for uninfected wounds or for clients who cannot tolerate sharp debridement.

7. One of the chief advantages of _____ dressings is that they allow the nurse to assess a wound without removing the dressing.

8. _____ are tubes that provide a means for removing blood and drainage from a wound.

9. _____ are knotted ties that hold an incision together that are generally constructed from silk or synthetic materials such as nylon.

10. A(n) _____ is a type of bandage generally applied to a particular body part such as the abdomen or breast.

Activity B *Consider the following figure.*

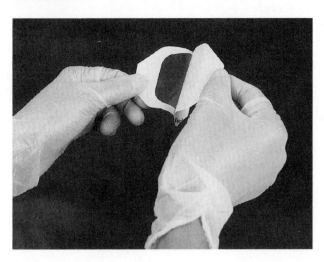

1. Identify the type of dressing.

   _____

   _____

   _____

2. What is the advantage of using this type of dressing?

   _____

   _____

   _____

Activity C *Match the terms related to wounds in column A with their description in column B.*

Column A

_____ **1.** Open wound

_____ **2.** Closed wound

_____ **3.** Granulation tissue

_____ **4.** First-intention healing

_____ **5.** Pressure ulcer

Column B

A. Occurs more often from blunt trauma or pressure

B. Wound caused by prolonged capillary compression

C. Surface of the skin or mucous membrane is no longer intact

D. A combination of new blood vessels, fibroblasts, and epithelial cells

E. A reparative process during which the wound edges are directly next to each other

Activity D *Presented here, in random order, are the stages of pressure ulcer development. Write the correct sequence in the boxes provided.*

1. Ulcer is red and accompanied by blistering or skin tear

2. Tissue is deeply ulcerated, exposing muscle and bone

3. Characterized by intact but reddened skin

4. Ulcer has a shallow skin crater that extends to the subcutaneous tissue

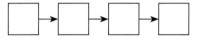

Activity E *Briefly answer the following.*

1. What is the purpose of inflammation during the process of wound repair?

   _____

   _____

   _____

2. How is the integrity of skin and damaged tissue restored?

   _____

   _____

   _____

3. What are the factors that affect wound healing?

   _____

   _____

   _____

4. What are the factors that affect blood flow to the injured tissue?

   _____

   _____

   _____

5. What are the possible causes of surgical wound complication?

_____

_____

_____

6. What purpose does the dressing of a wound serve?

_____

_____

_____

Activity F *Use the clues to complete the crossword puzzle.*

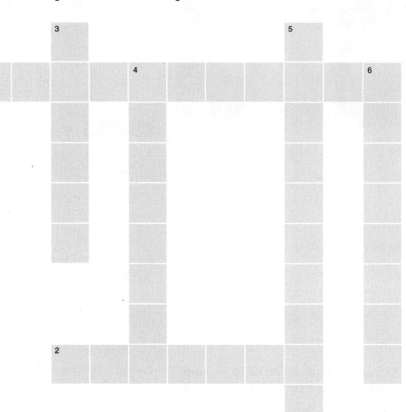

Across

1. Dressings that are self-adhesive, opaque, air-, and water-occlusive wound coverings
2. A strip or roll of cloth wrapped around the body part

Down

3. General term referring to injury
4. A tough inelastic protein substance
5. Moist, warm, or cool cloths that are applied to the skin
6. A cover over the wound

SECTION III: APPLYING YOUR KNOWLEDGE

Activity G *Heat and cold have various therapeutic uses and each can be used in several ways. Examples include an ice bag, collar, chemical pack, compress, and Aquathermia pad. Answer the following questions, which involve a nurse's role in the application of a compress.*

A nurse is caring for a 2-year-old-client who is being treated for viral fever at the health care facility. The nurse uses a cold compress for the child.

1. What is the purpose of a cold compress?

   _____

   _____

   _____

2. How should the nurse apply the compress to the client?

   _____

   _____

   _____

SECTION IV: PRACTICING FOR NCLEX

Activity H *Answer the following questions.*

1. The nurse is caring for a client with an open wound at the health care facility. The wound is a clean separation of skin and tissue with smooth, even edges. How should the nurse document this wound?
   a. Incision
   b. Abrasion
   c. Laceration
   d. Ulceration

2. A nurse is caring for a diabetic client with pressure ulcers on the sole of his feet. Which of the following best describes ulceration?
   a. A clean separation of skin and tissue with smooth, even edges
   b. A separation of skin and tissue in which the edges are torn and irregular

   c. A wound in which the surface layers of the skin are scraped away
   d. A shallow crater in which skin or mucous membrane is missing

3. A nurse is caring for a client who has an open wound in his leg caused by a cut from a piece of glass. Which of the following describes the inflammation stage of wound repair?
   a. Physiologic defense immediately after tissue injury
   b. The period during which new cells fill and seal the wound
   c. Process by which damaged cells recover and reestablish normal functioning
   d. The period during which the wound undergoes changes and maturation

4. A nurse is caring for a client who accidentally injured herself when using a knife. Which of the following actions take place first?
   a. Leukocytes, macrophages migrate to the injury site
   b. The body keeps producing white blood cells
   c. Increased neutrophils, monocytes
   d. Blood vessels constrict to control blood loss

5. A nurse is caring for a client with an open wound. Which of the following characteristics is indicative of a wound that heals by second intention?
   a. Wound edges are directly next to each other
   b. Wound edges are widely separated, leading to complex reparative process
   c. Wound edges are widely separated and brought together with closure material
   d. Wound edges are close to each other but require closure material

6. A nurse is caring for a client who has been confined to bed for a long time. During an assessment of the client's skin, the nurse observes redness accompanied by blistering or tears of skin. How should the nurse document this pressure ulcer?
   a. Stage I
   b. Stage II
   c. Stage III
   d. Stage IV

7. When caring for an elderly client, the nurse should remember that which of the following factors affect nutrition and consequently impair wound healing in older adults?

   a. Cognitive impairment

   b. Diminished collagen

   c. Decreased subcutaneous tissue

   d. Decreased blood supply

8. A nurse is treating an 11-year-old client who scraped his knee when he tripped and fell during a soccer match. The wound is bleeding and has some drainage. What type of dressing would be appropriate for this wound?

   a. Gauze

   b. Transparent

   c. Hydrocolloid

   d. Bandage

9. A nurse is caring for a client on intravenous therapy. The nurse uses a transparent dressing for the intravenous site. Which of the following is a benefit of using a transparent dressing?

   a. Occludes air and water from the wound

   b. Allows assessment of the wound without removing the dressing

   c. Allows treatment of wounds that are likely to bleed

   d. Keeps the wound moist, which promotes quick healing

10. A client who was severely injured with stab wounds has a closed suction drain. How should a nurse manage a closed drain site?

    a. Clean the insertion site in a circular manner

    b. Attach a safety pin or long clip

    c. Pull the drain for specified length

    d. Reposition a safety pin or long clip

11. A nurse is caring for a client with a superficial incision. What should the nurse use to manage the client's wound in this case?

    a. Hydrocolloid dressing

    b. Bandage

    c. Steri-Strips

    d. Gauze dressing

12. A nurse needs to bandage the arm of a client with a sprain resulting from a horse-riding accident. What techniques of wrapping the

roller bandage should the nurse use in this case?

    a. Spiral turn

    b. Figure-of-eight turn

    c. Spica turn

    d. Recurrent turn

13. A nurse uses the spica turn technique to bandage a client at the health care facility. For which of the following body parts would the nurse use this technique when bandaging a client?

    a. Elbow

    b. Legs

    c. Chest

    d. Knee

14. In which of the following cases would the nurse use the sharp debridement technique to promote healing?

    a. To treat clients with extensive necrotic tissue

    b. To treat clients with uninfected wounds

    c. To treat clients with small wounds

    d. To treat clients whose wounds are free of infection

15. A nurse is treating a 4-year-old with a solid object lodged in his ear. Before performing ear irrigation, the nurse performs a gross inspection of the client's ear. Which of the following reasons justify the nurse's intervention?

    a. The tapped object may swell and get more tightly fixed

    b. The pressure of the trapped solution could rupture the eardrum

    c. Drainage should be absorbed but should not obstruct its flow

    d. The tympanic membrane may become perforated

16. The nurse at the health care facility is caring for an 80-year-old client whose tests show reduced T-lymphocyte cells. The nurse should be aware that diminished immune response from reduced T-lymphocyte cells predisposes older adults to which of the following?

    a. Pressure ulcers

    b. Shear-type injuries

    c. Delayed healing

    d. Wound infection

CHAPTER 29

Gastrointestinal Intubation

SECTION I: LEARNING OBJECTIVES

- Define intubation.
- List six reasons for gastrointestinal intubation.
- Identify four general types of gastrointestinal tubes.
- Name at least four assessments that are necessary before inserting a tube nasally.
- Explain the purpose of and how to obtain a NEX measurement.
- Describe three techniques for checking distal placement in the stomach.
- Discuss three ways that nasointestinal feeding tubes or their insertion differ from their gastric counterparts.
- Name two common problems associated with transabdominal tubes.
- Define enteral nutrition.
- Name four schedules for administering tube feedings.
- Explain the purpose for assessing gastric residual.
- Name five nursing activities involved in managing the care of clients who are being tube-fed.
- List four items of information to include in the written instructions for clients administering their own tube feedings.
- Name two nursing responsibilities for assisting with the insertion of a tungsten-weighted intestinal decompression tube.

SECTION II: ASSESSING YOUR UNDERSTANDING

Activity A *Fill in the blanks.*

1. A(n) _____ is an artificial opening into the stomach.

2. Gastric _____ tubes are used exclusively to remove fluid and gas from the stomach.

3. Belching often indicates that the tip of the tube is still in the _____.

4. A(n) _____ decompression tube is inserted in the same manner as a nasogastric tube.

5. Intestinal tubes like the Maxter tube are now weighted with _____.

6. A(n) _____ tube is used in an emergency to remove toxic substances that have been ingested.

7. Some nasogastric tubes have more than one _____ within the tube.

8. A gastrostomy tube is placed surgically or with the use of a(n) _____.

9. A(n) _____ feeding usually involves 250 to 400 mL formula per administration.

10. _____ generally means the placement of a tube into a body structure.

Activity B *Consider the following figures.*

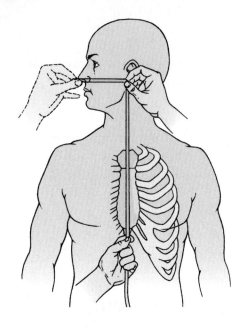

1. Identify the image.

_____

_____

_____

2. How is this procedure done?

_____

_____

_____

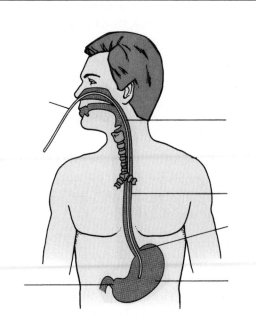

3. Identify and label the image.

_____

_____

_____

4. What are the disadvantages of this procedure?

_____

_____

_____

Activity C *Match the type of liquid nutrition in column A with its use in column B.*

Column A

_____ **1.** Balanced

_____ **2.** High nitrogen

_____ **3.** High fiber

_____ **4.** Partially hydrolyzed

_____ **5.** Isotonic balanced

Column B

A. Given to people with malabsorption syndromes

B. Meets total nutrition needs

C. Furnishes more protein than other formulas

D. Provides nutrition and decreases constipation or diarrhea

E. Supplements nutrition without altering water distribution

Activity D *Presented here, in random order, are steps that occur during the assessment of the pH of aspirated fluid. Write the correct sequence in the boxes provided.*

1. Aspirate a small volume of fluid with a clean syringe.

2. Perform an alcohol-based hand rub.

3. Compare the color on the test strip with color guide.

4. Drop a sample of gastric fluid onto an indicator strip.

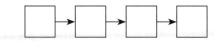

Activity E *Briefly answer the following.*

1. Why is intubation performed on clients?

_____

_____

_____

2. What are the problems faced with narrow-diameter feeding tubes?

_____

_____

_____

3. What are the nurse's functions regarding naso-gastric tubes?

_____

_____

_____

4. When are tube feedings performed?

_____

_____

5. What are the problems associated with bolus feedings?

_____

_____

6. How can a dietitian help a tube-fed client in a home setting?

_____

_____

Activity F *Use the clues to complete the crossword puzzle.*

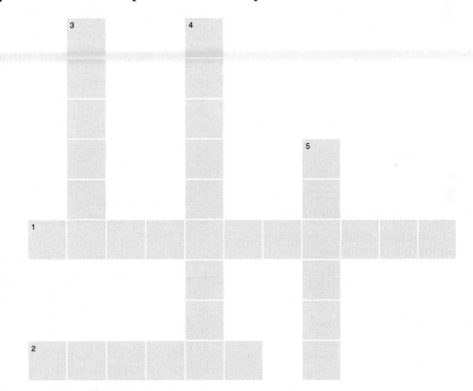

Across

1. A transabdominal tube that leads to the small intestine
2. A metal guidewire that helps to straighten feeding tubes

Down

3. Process of forced feeding by stomach tube
4. Process of controlling gastric bleeding with pressure
5. A surgically created opening for the insertion of a tube

SECTION III: APPLYING YOUR KNOWLEDGE

Activity G *Older adults are at an increased risk of fluid and electrolyte disturbances and, as a result, may develop hyperglycemia when tube feedings are administered. Most tube-feeding formulas are highly concentrated; therefore, the hydration status of the older client must be closely monitored. Answer the following questions, which involve the nurse's role in caring for a client undergoing tube feeding.*

A nurse is administering a tube-feeding formula to an elderly client with severe abdominal pain. The client also experiences malabsorption syndromes.

1. What should the nurse do if the elderly client develops hyperglycemia when tube-feeding?

   _____

   _____

   _____

2. Which tube-feed formula should the nurse administer to the elderly client?

   _____

   _____

   _____

SECTION IV: PRACTICING FOR NCLEX

Activity H *Answer the following questions.*

1. A nurse has to administer liquid nourishment to a client over 30 to 60 minutes at the rate of 250 to 400 mL per administration with a feeding pump. Which of the following tube-feeding cycles should the nurse follow?
   a. Intermittent feeding
   b. Cyclic feeding
   c. Continuous feeding
   d. Bolus feeding

2. A nurse needs to insert a nasointestinal tube inside the nostril of a client. Which of the following should the nurse ask the client to perform when assessing each nostril?
   a. Use a nebulizer for half an hour
   b. Perform presurgical skin preparation
   c. Avoid clearing nasal debris
   d. Ask the client to exhale

3. A nurse has to insert an intestinal decompression tube from the pyloric valve into the small intestine of a client. Which of following actions should the nurse perform?
   a. Observe the graduated marks on the tube
   b. Move the client into the Fowler's position
   c. Ambulate the client if possible
   d. Request an X-ray confirmation

4. A nurse has to remove an intestinal decompression tube from a client. Which of the following actions should the nurse perform first when removing an intestinal decompression tube?
   a. Remove the tube within 10 minutes
   b. Disconnect the tube from the suction source
   c. Secure the tube to the face with tape
   d. Verify the tube placement with a radiograph

5. A nurse is performing a preintubation assessment for a client who has been prescribed a nasogastric tube. Which of the following is the main goal of the assessment?
   a. Determine whether there is any nausea and vomiting
   b. Determine the client's ability to swallow, cough, and gag
   c. Detect the nostril best suited for tube insertion
   d. Check the client's level of consciousness

6. A nurse is inserting a gastric sump tube inside a client. Which of the following activities is most suitable with the use of a gastric sump tube?
   a. Removes fluid and gas from the stomach
   b. Provides nourishment to the small intestine
   c. Removes liquid contents from the small intestine
   d. Reduces trauma to intestinal tissue

7. A nurse is caring for a client who is provided with liquid nourishment on a cyclic feeding schedule. Which of the following times is most suitable for tube-feeding the client?
   a. Early morning
   b. Afternoon
   c. Late evening
   d. After lunch

8. A nurse is checking the gastric residual of a client who is being tube-fed. As a rule of thumb, how much should the volume of gastric residual be?
   a. Less than 250 mL
   b. Approximately 150 mL
   c. 1 mL/kcal, on a daily basis
   d. No more than 100 mL

9. A physician has ordered a nurse to provide enteral nutrition to a client. Which of the following actions should the nurse perform to provide enteral nutrition? Select all that apply.
   a. Provide nourishment via the stomach
   b. Administer a liquid tube-feeding formula
   c. Provide nourishment via the intestine
   d. Use a tube that is short in length
   e. Use a tube that is small in diameter

10. A nurse is preparing a home care note for a tube-fed client who is being discharged from the health care facility. Which of the following points is most important when preparing clients to take care of themselves at home?
    a. Demonstrate each procedure
    b. Provide detailed written instructions
    c. Make a referral to a home health agency
    d. Teach self-administration techniques

11. A nurse is inserting an intestinal decompression tube inside a client. Which of the following actions will help the nurse to monitor the tube's progression and approximate anatomic location?
    a. Observe graduated marks on the tube
    b. Reinsert the stylet when the tube is inside
    c. Ambulate the client if possible
    d. Mark the tube before inserting

12. A nurse is assessing a feeding tube smaller than 12 Fr, which is prone to obstruction. Which of the following actions should the nurse perform to maintain tube patency? Select all that apply.
    a. Wash the tube every 2 hours
    b. Give plenty of water to the client
    c. Flush the tube with 30 to 60 mL water
    d. Flush the tube with cranberry juice
    e. Flush the tube with carbonated beverages

13. A nurse has to tube-feed a client. Which of the following tube-feeding schedules is least desirable because it distends the stomach rapidly, causes gastric discomfort, and increases risk of reflux?
    a. Continuous
    b. Bolus
    c. Intermittent
    d. Cyclic

14. A nurse is rectifying a gastrostomy leak that has occurred in a feeding tube inserted in a client. Which of the following are causes of a gastrostomy leak? Select all that apply.
    a. Infusion of the feed when the gastrointestinal tube is clamped
    b. Reduction in abdominal pressure
    c. Disconnection between the feeding tube and the gastrointestinal tube
    d. Instillation of highly concentrated nutritional formula
    e. Underinflation of the balloon beneath the skin

15. A client with a nasogastric tube complains of a vomiting sensation. The nurse assesses the client and notices that the client's bowel sounds are less than five per minute. Which of the following nursing diagnoses should the nurse document based on the data collected during client care?
    a. Imbalanced nutrition
    b. Self-care deficit
    c. Impaired swallowing
    d. Risk for aspiration

16. A nurse is administering a tube feeding to a client. The nurse pinches the feeding tube just as the last volume of water is administered. Which of the following reasons is most appropriate for the nurse's action?

    a. To provide access to formula

    b. To prevent the tube from leaking

    c. To prevent air from entering the tube

    d. To purge air from the tube

17. A nurse is caring for a tube-fed client who has inflammation of the middle ear. Which of the following nursing interventions will reduce the inflammation?

    a. Insert a small-diameter feeding tube

    b. Provide nasal and oral hygiene

    c. Keep the tubing filled with water

    d. Maintain the client's neck in a neutral position

CHAPTER 30

Urinary Elimination

SECTION I: LEARNING OBJECTIVES

- Identify the collective functions of the urinary system.
- Name at least five factors that affect urination.
- List four physical characteristics of urine.
- Name four types of urine specimens that nurses commonly collect.
- List six abnormal urinary elimination patterns.
- Identify three alternative devices for urinary elimination.
- Define continence training.
- Name three types of urinary catheters.
- Describe two principles that apply to using a closed drainage system.
- Explain why catheter care is important in the nursing management of clients with retention catheters.
- Discuss the purpose for irrigating a catheter.
- Identify three ways of irrigating a catheter.
- Define urinary diversion.
- Discuss factors that contribute to impaired skin integrity in clients with a urostomy.
- Describe two age-related changes in older adults that may affect urinary elimination.

SECTION II: ASSESSING YOUR UNDERSTANDING

Activity A *Fill in the blanks.*

1. A(n) _____ specimen is a sample of fresh urine collected in a clean container.

2. _____ means the absence of urine or a urinary volume of 100 mL or less in 24 hours.

3. In _____ the urine output is less than 400 mL per 24 hours, which indicates the inadequate elimination of urine.

4. _____ is difficult or uncomfortable voiding and a common symptom of trauma to the urethra or a bladder infection.

5. _____ refers to using a device inside the bladder or externally about the urinary meatus.

6. A(n) _____ catheter is a urine drainage tube inserted, but not left in place; it drains urine temporarily or provides a sterile urine specimen.

7. A(n) _____ irrigation instills irrigating solution into a catheter by gravity over a period of days.

8. Age-related changes, such as diminished bladder capacity and relaxation of the pelvic floor muscle tone, increase the risk of _____.

9. A(n) _____ catheter is not inserted within the bladder; instead, it surrounds the urinary meatus.

10. A(n) _____ is a seatlike container for elimination that is used to collect urine or stool.

Activity B *Consider the following figure.*

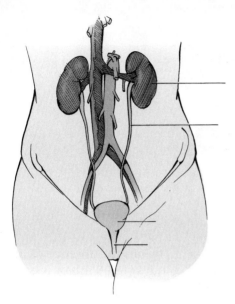

1. Identify and label the figure.

   _____

   _____

   _____

2. What are the functions of these structures?

   _____

   _____

   _____

Activity C *Match the terms related to urinary elimination in column A with their description in column B.*

Column A

_____ **1.** Urinary elimination

_____ **2.** Clean catch

_____ **3.** Polyuria

_____ **4.** Urinal

_____ **5.** Catheter irrigation

Column B

A. Voided sample of urine that is considered sterile

B. Cylindrical container for collecting urine

C. Technique for restoring or maintaining catheter patency

D. Process of releasing excess of fluid and metabolic waste

E. Greater-than-normal urinary volume and may accompany minor dietary variations

Activity D *Presented here, in random order, are steps that occur when providing a continuous irrigation. Write the correct sequence in the boxes provided.*

1. Connect the tubing to the catheter port for irrigation.

2. Monitor the appearance of the urine and volume of urinary drainage.

3. Purge the air from the tubing.

4. Regulate the rate of infusion according to the medical order.

5. Hang the sterile irrigating solution from an intravenous pole.

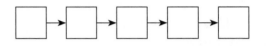

Activity E *Briefly answer the following.*

1. What are the common disorders associated with polyuria?

   _____

   _____

   _____

2. What is a urinary catheter used for?

   _____

   _____

   _____

3. What are the problems that may accompany the use of a condom catheter?

   _____

   _____

   _____

4. What physiologic changes could lead older adults to experience urinary urgency and frequency?

   _____

   _____

   _____

5. What are the resources available to assist older adults in evaluating and treating incontinence?

_____

_____

_____

6. What are the problems that a client with oliguria is likely to face?

_____

_____

_____

Activity F *Use the clues to complete the crossword puzzle.*

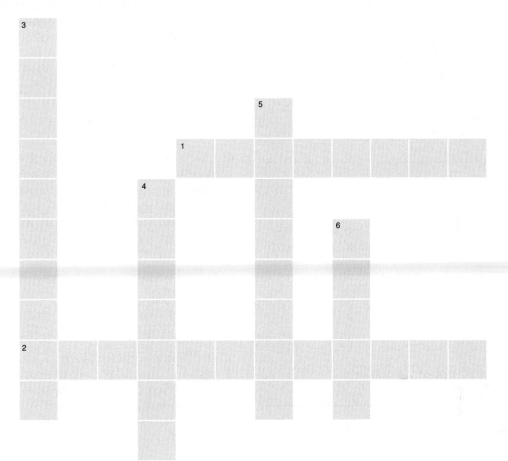

Across

1. Urinary diversion that discharges urine from an opening in the abdomen
2. Inability to control either urinary or bowel elimination

Down

3. Urine containing glucose
4. Chair with an opening in the seat under which a receptacle is placed
5. Nighttime urination
6. A common type of retention catheter

SECTION III: APPLYING YOUR KNOWLEDGE

Activity G *A closed drainage system is a device used to collect urine from a catheter. It consists of a calibrated bag that can be opened at the bottom, tubing of sufficient length to accommodate the turning and positioning of clients, and a hanger from which to suspend the bag from the bed. Answer the following questions related to the use of a closed drainage system.*

A nurse is caring for a client with a urinary catheter at the health care facility. The client has a distended bladder and is unable to void.

1. What care should the nurse take when a closed drainage system is used to collect urine from the catheter?

   _____

   _____

   _____

2. How can the nurse prevent the drainage system from becoming a reservoir of pathogens?

   _____

   _____

   _____

SECTION IV: PRACTICING FOR NCLEX

Activity H *Answer the following questions.*

1. Order the following steps on how the need to urinate becomes apparent.
   a. Distention with urine causes increased fluid pressure.
   b. This creates a desire to urinate.
   c. The bladder distends with 150 to 300 mL urine.
   d. This stimulates the stretch receptors in the bladder wall.

2. When collecting a clean-catch urine specimen, what can the nurse do to prevent the urine sample from being contaminated by

microorganisms or substances other than those in the urine?
   a. Collect the sample in a clean container
   b. Clean external structures through which the urine passes
   c. Collect the sample over a period of 24 hours
   d. Use a catheter to collect the sample

3. A nurse at the health care facility notes that the volume of the client's urine is more than 3,500 mL/day. Which of the following could have led to the increase in volume of the client's urine?
   a. Kidney dysfunction
   b. Gallbladder disease
   c. Diuretic medication
   d. Infection

4. A nurse at the health care facility needs to collect a sample of the client's urine. However, when collecting the sample, the nurse notes that the client's urine appears cloudy. Which of the following is the possible reason for the appearance of the urine?
   a. Stasis
   b. Blood
   c. Water-soluble dyes
   d. Dehydration

5. The laboratory test of a client's urine indicates the presence of plasma proteins in the urine. What term could the nurse use to document this type of urine?
   a. Hematuria
   b. Pyuria
   c. Proteinuria
   d. Albuminuria

6. An assessment of a client's urinary pattern indicates that the client has dysuria. Which of the following is indicative of dysuria?
   a. Absence of urine
   b. Inadequate elimination of urine
   c. Greater-than-normal urinary volume
   d. Difficult or uncomfortable voiding

7. The abnormal urinary elimination pattern in a client has been diagnosed as oliguria. Which of the following problems are commonly seen in client's with oliguria?

   a. Urinary stones

   b. Diabetes mellitus

   c. Diabetes insipidus

   d. Enlarged prostate gland

8. When caring for male clients at the health care facility who require assistance with urinary elimination, for which of the following clients should the nurse use a urinal?

   a. Clients who can ambulate

   b. Clients who are weak

   c. Clients who are unable to walk

   d. Clients who are confined to bed

9. The nurse at the health care facility is caring for a client with urinary incontinence. The client has been provided with a catheter. For what purposes is a catheter used for a client? Select all that apply.

   a. Restraining the client from urinating

   b. Keeping the incontinent client dry

   c. Measuring the residual urine

   d. Instilling medication within the bladder

   e. Preventing urinary tract infection

10. A nurse uses a urinary bag to collect a urine specimen from an infant at the health care facility. Which of the following statements describes a urinary bag?

    a. A urine drainage tube inserted but not left in place

    b. A urine drainage tube that is left in place over a period of time

    c. A bag attached by adhesive backing to the skin around genitals

    d. A flexible sheath that is rolled around the penis

11. A nurse is caring for a client who complains of the loss of a small amount of urine whenever she sneezes or laughs. What nursing intervention should the nurse suggest for this client?

    a. Clothing modification

    b. Weight reduction

    c. Absorbent undergarment

    d. Cutaneous triggering

12. A client with urge incontinence complains to the nurse that the she perceives the need to void frequently and has a short-lived ability to sustain control of the flow. What is the possible cause of the client's condition?

    a. Loss of perineal and sphincter muscle tone

    b. Damage to the motor and sensory tracts in the lower spinal cord

    c. Altered consciousness related to head injury

    d. Bladder irritation secondary to infection

13. A nurse is caring for a client who has a retention catheter for urinary incontinence. When providing catheter care, why should the nurse clean the meatus and nearby section of the catheter at least once a day?

    a. To reduce the colonizing of microorganisms

    b. To remove gross secretions and transient microorganisms

    c. To protect the bed linen from becoming wet or soiled

    d. To reduce the potential for transmitting microorganisms

14. Order the following steps on irrigating a closed drainage system.

    a. Attach a needle to the syringe containing the sterile irrigation solution.

    b. Clean the port with an alcohol swab.

    c. Clamp the tubing beneath the port and instill the solution.

    d. Pierce the port with an 18- or 19-guage 1.5 inch needle.

    e. Release the tubing for drainage.

15. Order the following steps with regard to providing continuous irrigation.

    a. Hang the sterile irrigating solution from an intravenous pole.

    b. Regulate the rate of infusion according to the medical order.

    c. Purge the air from the tubing.

    d. Monitor the appearance of the urine and volume of urinary drainage.

    e. Connect the tubing to the catheter port for irrigation.

16. When caring for an elderly client at the health care facility, the nurse should understand that which of the following conditions could increase the risk for a urinary tract infection in the client?

    a. Diminished bladder capacity

    b. Pelvic floor muscle tone relaxation

    c. Chronic residual urine

    d. Enlargement of the prostate

17. A nurse at the health care facility teaches double voiding to a client who is being treated for urinary tract infection resulting from residual urine. Which of the following statements describe double voiding?

    a. Clients void then wait a few more minutes to allow any urine to be voided

    b. Clients void within 30 to 120 minutes after medication administration

    c. Clients plan toilet breaks every 60 to 90 minutes

    d. Clients have a routine toileting schedule every 90 to 120 minutes

18. A nurse provides a bedpan to a client who has been confined to the bed. Before using the pan, the nurse palpates the lower abdomen. Which of the following statements justifies the nurse's action?

    a. Demonstrates concern for the client's comfort

    b. Prevents unnecessary exposure

    c. Promotes use of good body mechanics

    d. Checks for bladder fullness

19. When collecting a urine sample from the client for laboratory tests, the nurse notes that the client's urine appears dark amber in color. Which is following is the possible cause for the appearance of the urine?

    a. Dehydration

    b. Liver disease

    c. Blood

    d. Water-soluble dyes

CHAPTER 31

Bowel Elimination

SECTION I: LEARNING OBJECTIVES

- Describe the process of defecation.
- Name two components of a bowel elimination assessment.
- List five common alterations in bowel elimination.
- Name four types of constipation.
- Identify measures within the scope of nursing practice for treating constipation.
- Identify two interventions that promote bowel elimination when it does not occur naturally.
- Name two categories of enema administration.
- List at least three common solutions used in a cleansing enema.
- Explain the purpose of an oil retention enema.
- Name four nursing activities involved in ostomy care.

SECTION II: ASSESSING YOUR UNDERSTANDING

Activity A *Fill in the blanks.*

1. _____ is the rhythmic contractions of intestinal smooth muscle that facilitate defecation.

2. _____ is eventually released when the anal sphincters relax.

3. _____ is an elimination problem characterized by dry, hard stool that is difficult to pass.

4. The incidence of constipation tends to be high among those whose dietary habits lack adequate _____.

5. Prolonged use of narcotic analgesia tends to cause _____ constipation.

6. Clients with a fecal _____ usually report a frequent desire to defecate but an inability to do so.

7. _____ results from swallowing air while eating or sluggish peristalsis.

8. A(n) _____ enema holds a solution within the large intestine for a specified period.

9. _____ constipation is a consequence of a pathologic disorder such as a partial bowel obstruction.

10. Dietary fiber that becomes undigested cellulose attracts _____ within the bowel.

Activity B *Consider the following figure.*

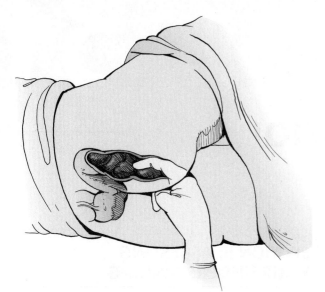

1. Identify the image.

   _____

   _____

   _____

2. When is the procedure required?

   _____

   _____

   _____

Activity C *Match the factors affecting bowel elimination in column A with their effects in column B.*

Column A

____ **1.** Types of food consumed

____ **2.** Fluid intake

____ **3.** Neuromuscular function

____ **4.** Abdominal muscle tone

____ **5.** Opportunity for defecation

Column B

A. Inhibits or facilitates elimination

B. Influence color, odor, and volume

C. Influences moisture content of stool

D. Ability to control rectal muscles

E. Ability to increase intra-abdominal pressure

Activity D *Presented here, in random order, are steps that occur during the procedure of testing stool for occult blood. Write the correct sequence in the boxes provided.*

1. Take the sample from the center of the stool.

2. Place two drops of chemical agent onto the test space.

3. Collect stool within a toilet line or bedpan.

4. Apply a thin smear of stool onto the test area.

5. Wait for 60 seconds and observe the blue color.

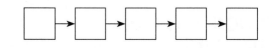

Activity E *Briefly answer the following.*

1. What problems do clients with musculoskeletal disorders face?

   _____

   _____

   _____

2. What is defecation?

   _____

   _____

   _____

3. What is involved in a comprehensive assessment of bowel elimination?

   _____

   _____

   _____

4. Which are the common problems faced by clients in bowel elimination?

   _____

   _____

   _____

5. How does a client develop pseudoconstipation?

_____

_____

_____

6. What is diarrhea?

_____

_____

_____

Activity F *Use the clues to complete the crossword puzzle.*

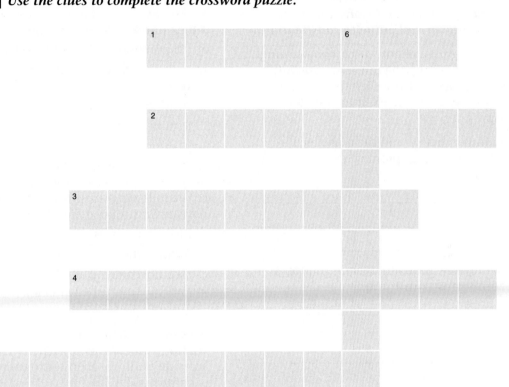

Across

1. They alter bowel motility
2. It is a surgically created opening to a portion of the colon
3. It is a surgically created opening to the ileum
4. Chemical injury of skin caused by enzymes in stool
5. They ease insertion

Down

6. Another term used for persons with an ostomy

SECTION III: APPLYING YOUR KNOWLEDGE

Activity G *Infrequent elimination of stool does not necessarily indicate that a person is constipated. Some people may be constipated even though they have a daily bowel movement, whereas others who defecate irregularly may have normal bowel function. Answer the following questions, which involve the nurse's role when caring for a client with constipation.*

A nurse is caring for a client who is complaining of constipation. During the initial assessment, the nurse finds out that the client has a sedentary job and eats convenience store food for lunch and dinner.

1. What kind of diet should the nurse recommend to the client to promote quick and easy elimination?

   _____

   _____

   _____

2. Which are the various signs and symptoms that accompany constipation?

   _____

   _____

   _____

SECTION IV: PRACTICING FOR NCLEX

Activity H *Answer the following questions.*

1. A nurse is caring for a client with abnormal stool. The nurse knows that abnormal stool can appear in which of the following colors? Select all that apply.
   a. Black
   b. Green
   c. Brown
   d. Yellow
   e. Dark brown

2. A nurse is caring for a client with severe pain in the abdomen and constipation resulting from fecal impaction. Which of the following interventions should the nurse perform to facilitate easy insertion within the rectum when removing the fecal impaction?
   a. Lubricate the forefinger
   b. Place the client in the Sims' position
   c. Lubricate the rectal tube
   d. Warm the cleansing solution

3. A nurse is caring for a client with fecal impaction accompanied by rectal pain. The nurse knows that the rectal pain is the result of which of the following factors?
   a. Contractions in higher bowel areas
   b. Unsuccessful efforts to empty the lower bowel
   c. Insufficient intake of liquids
   d. Retained barium from a radiographic procedure

4. A nurse is caring for a client who is extremely uncomfortable because of flatulence. Which of the following nursing interventions can provide immediate relief to the client?
   a. Insertion of a rectal suppository
   b. Administration of a cleansing enema
   c. Insertion of a rectal tube
   d. Offering a glass of prune juice

5. A nurse is caring for a client with an intestinal disorder. Which of the following interventions should the nurse perform to get accurate findings when testing the stool for occult blood?
   a. Avoid placing reagent onto the test space
   b. Cover the entire test space with the sample
   c. Apply a thin smear of stool onto test area
   d. Avoid taking the sample from the center of the stool

6. A physician has asked the nurse to include a power pudding recipe in an elderly client's diet. Which of the following ingredients should the nurse incorporate in the power pudding recipe? Select all that apply.
   a. One cup prune juice
   b. One cup applesauce
   c. One cup of milk
   d. One cup wheat bran
   e. One cup water

7. A physician has ordered the nurse to increase the fluid intake in a client's diet. What will be the effect of increased liquid intake on the client's bowel elimination?

a. Influence the odor and volume of stool

b. Alter the bowel motility

c. Influence the moisture content of stool

d. Influence the fecal velocity

8. A nurse is removing the fecal impaction of a client. Which of the following actions should the nurse perform to facilitate digital manipulation of the stool?

a. Move the finger slowly and carefully

b. Place the client in the Sims' position

c. Lubricate and insert the finger periodically

d. Insert the finger to the level of the hardened mass

9. A nurse is administering a water and soap solution enema to a client. Which of the following steps should the nurse perform to purge air from the tubing?

a. Open the clamp and fill the tube with solution

b. Hold the solution container 20 inches above the client's anus

c. Lubricate the tip of the tube generously

d. Instill the solution gradually over 5 to 10 minutes

10. A nurse is caring for a client with constipation related to inadequate dietary habits. Which of the following food items should the nurse encourage the client to eat to promote hydration and avoid dry stool? Select all that apply.

a. Prune juice

b. Apple juice

c. Oral fluids

d. Banana pulp

e. Cottage cheese

11. A nurse is administering a prescribed cleansing enema to a client with colitis. Which of the following consequences can occur if the nurse administers a large-volume cleansing enema to a client?

a. Increase the fecal velocity

b. Rupture the bowel

c. Irritate the local tissue

d. Draw fluid from body tissue

12. A physician has ordered the nurse to administer an oil retention enema to a client for easier expulsion. For how long should the nurse ask the client to retain the cleansing solution within the large intestine?

a. At least 1 hour

b. At least 10 minutes

c. At least 5 minutes

d. At least half an hour

13. A nurse is assessing an elderly client who is overly self-conscious of her poor bowel elimination habits. Which of the following habits can instill healthy elimination habits in older adults?

a. Avoid high-fiber products like polycarbophil

b. Increase dosage of laxatives gradually

c. Use bulk-forming products with psyllium

d. Use mineral oil retention enemas regularly

14. A nurse is assessing a client for fecal impaction. Which of the following assessments aptly indicate that the client has fecal impaction?

a. The client passes liquid stool frequently

b. The client has foul breath

c. The client has lost weight drastically

d. The client has poor physical reflexes

15. A nurse is administering prescribed medicine to a client with diarrhea. Which of the following factors can lead to diarrhea? Select all that apply.

a. Poor fluid intake

b. Laxative abuse

c. Physical inactivity

d. Bowel disorder

e. Emotional stress

16. A nurse is digitally removing the hardened mass of stool from the rectum of a client. Why is it important for the nurse to remove the impaction gently?

a. To prevent bleeding and tissue trauma

b. To preserve the client's dignity and self-esteem

c. To develop healthy bowel elimination

d. To provide privacy and prevent soiling

32

Oral Medications

SECTION I: LEARNING OBJECTIVES

- Define the term *medication.*
- Name seven components of a drug order.
- Explain the difference between trade and generic drug names.
- Name four common routes for administration.
- Describe the oral route and two general forms of medication administered this way.
- Explain the purpose of a medication record.
- Name three ways that drugs are supplied.
- Discuss two nursing responsibilities that apply to the administration of narcotics.
- Name the five rights of medication administration.
- Give the formula for calculating a drug dose.
- Discuss at least one guideline that applies to the safe administration of medications.
- Discuss one point to stress when teaching clients about taking medications.
- Explain the circumstances involved in giving oral medications by an enteral tube and one commonly associated problem.
- Describe three appropriate actions in the event of a medication error.

SECTION II: ASSESSING YOUR UNDERSTANDING

Activity A *Fill in the blanks.*

1. Medications are _____ substances that change body function.

2. A(n) _____ tablet is convenient when only part of a tablet is needed.

3. _____ orders are instructions for client care that are given during face-to-face conversations.

4. _____ blood albumin levels increase the active drug components for protein-bound medications.

5. Older people taking more than one medication are more likely to develop _____ changes as an early and common sign of adverse effects.

6. _____ therapists are helpful in evaluating dysphagia and recommending safe and effective methods of administering oral medications.

7. _____ name is the chemical name not protected by a company's trademark.

8. The oral route facilitates drug absorption through the _____ tract.

9. A(n) _____ supply remains on the nursing unit for use in an emergency or so that a nurse can give a drug without delay.

10. The nurse accesses the computerized system by using a(n) _____ and then selects the appropriate choice from a computerized menu.

Activity B *Consider the following figure.*

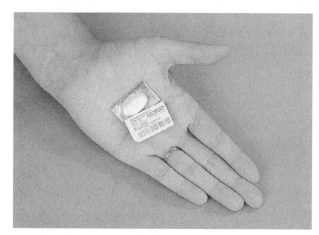

1. Identify the figure shown here.

_____

_____

2. What is the purpose of this method of supply-ing medications?

_____

_____

_____

Activity C *Match the terms related with oral medication in column A with their descriptions in column B.*

Column A

_____ **1.** Trade name

_____ **2.** Oral route

_____ **3.** Enteric-coated tablets

_____ **4.** Medication administration record

_____ **5.** Pill organizer

Column B

A. Administration of drugs by swallowing or instillation through an enteral tube

B. A simple-to-use medication man-agement system

C. Agency form used to document drug administration

D. Used by the phar-maceutical company who made the drug

E. Solid drug covered with a substance that dissolves beyond the stomach

Activity D *Briefly answer the following.*

1. What is meant by frequency of drug adminis-tration?

_____

_____

_____

2. What are the components of a medical order?

_____

_____

_____

3. What is the importance of health teaching with regard to the administration of medication?

_____

_____

_____

4. Why is the client's medication not added to the formula during tube feeding?

_____

_____

_____

5. How does the computerized documentation of medication help at the health care agency?

_____

_____

_____

6. What should the nurse do when a medication error occurs?

_____

_____

_____

Activity E *Use the clues to complete the crossword puzzle.*

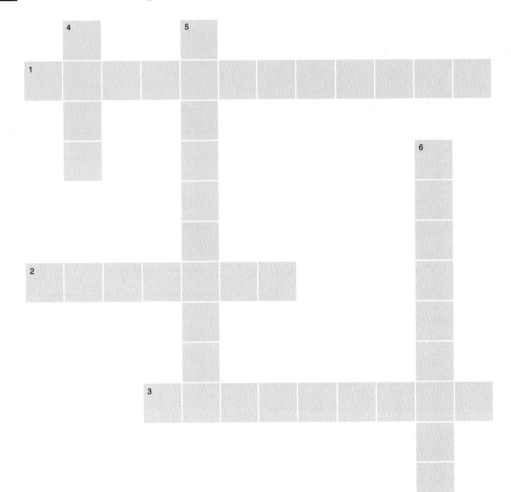

Across

1. Administration of multiple medications to the same person
2. Method of administration of medication by application to the skin or mucous membrane
3. Swallowing difficulties

Down

4. The amount of a drug to administer
5. Measurements that may be subject to future exclusion because they are unfamiliar to many practitioners
6. Federal law regulates their possession and administration

SECTION III: APPLYING YOUR KNOWLEDGE

Activity F *One of the nurse's most important responsibilities is the administration of medications. Providing health teaching helps to ensure that clients administer their own medications safely and remain compliant. Answer the following questions related to health teaching regarding the administration of medication.*

A nurse is providing health teaching with regard to the administration of medication for an elderly client who is being discharged from the health care facility.

1. What should the nurse do if the elderly client is having difficulty comprehending information about the medication routines?

   _____

   _____

   _____

2. What should the nurse include in the health teaching for this client?

   _____

   _____

   _____

SECTION IV: PRACTICING FOR NCLEX

Activity G *Answer the following questions.*

1. A client has been admitted to the health care facility with complaints of abdominal pains. Under what condition would the nurse be permitted to write a medication order?
   a. If the nurse is a registered nurse
   b. If it is permitted by the health care facility
   c. If the nurse has a baccalaureate degree
   d. If it is legally permitted by the state's statutes

2. A physician prepares a medication order for a client who is being treated for chickenpox. The nurse should be aware that which of the following components form a part of a valid medication order? Select all that apply.
   a. Name of the client
   b. Age of the client
   c. Dose to be administered
   d. Route of administration
   e. Name of the primary nurse

3. A nurse administers medication to the client per the medication order prepared by the physician. The medication order contains the trade name of the drug. The nurse knows that the chemical name of the drug that is not protected by the company's trademark is known as which of the following?
   a. Trade name
   b. Proprietary name
   c. Generic name
   d. Brand name

4. A nurse needs to administer medication through the oral route to a client with influenza. Which of the following methods of administration is the oral route?
   a. Administration of the drug by swallowing
   b. Administration of the drug by application on the skin
   c. Administration of the drug through an aerosol
   d. Administration of the drug by injections

5. Per the physician's medication order, a client needs to be administered half a tablet three times a day. The nurse knows that which of the following types of solid medication would allow this type of administration?
   a. Enteric-coated tablets
   b. Scored tablets
   c. Sustained-release capsules
   d. Pellets

6. Per the physician's medication orders, the nurse needs to administer a particular drug four times a day. What standard abbreviation would the physician use in this case?

a. q4h

b. b.i.d.

c. t.i.d.

d. q.i.d.

7. A physician at the health care facility orders a "qh" administration of medication to a client who is critically ill. What is the frequency of administration of the medication?

a. Immediately

b. Every day

c. Hourly

d. Twice a day

8. A physician dictates the medication order to a nurse over the telephone. What should the nurse do to ensure the accuracy of the medication order? Select all that apply.

a. Repeat the dosage of drugs

b. Spell the drug name for confirmation

c. Write "V.O." at the end of the order

d. Write down the order on a note pad

e. Have a second nurse listen simultaneously

9. A nurse at the health care facility requests the drugs from the pharmacy once the medication order has been transcribed to the MAR. The nurse uses the individual supply method to dispense medication. What is an individual supply of medications?

a. Contains enough prescribed drugs for several days

b. Holds one tablet or capsule for individual clients

c. Remains on the nursing unit for use in emergency

d. Contains frequently used medication for that unit

10. A physician at the health care facility prescribes morphine for a client. What are the responsibilities of the nurse with regard to the administration of narcotic medication? Select all that apply.

a. Have an accurate account of their use

b. Keep them on the nursing unit for emergency

c. Record each narcotic used from stock supply

d. Place it in the container with prescribed drugs

e. Count each narcotic at the change of each shift

11. A nurse at the health care facility needs to administer prescribed drugs to a client at the health care facility. What precaution should the nurse take before, during, and after every administration to avoid potential medication errors?

a. Calculate the drug dosage accurately per the medication order

b. Request a second nurse to confirm the drug dosage calculation

c. Ask the physician to mention the dosage in the medication order

d. Count the number of drugs that has been supplied

12. Per the physician's medication order, the nurse needs to administer 250 mg of the drug to the client orally, three times a day. However, the drug is available in 500 mg/5 mL. What quantity of the drug should the nurse administer to the client?

a. 5.5 mL

b. 2.5 mL

c. 1.5 mL

d. 7.5 mL

13. A nurse at the health care facility prepares the drug dosage to be administered to the client. Before administering the drugs to the client, why should the nurse compare the MAR with the written medical order?

a. Avoids potential complication

b. Ensures appropriate administration

c. Demonstrates compliance with the medical order

d. Prevents medication errors

14. The nurse needs to administer medication through an enteral tube for a client who has difficulty swallowing medication through the mouth. When administering the medication, the nurse interrupts the tube feeding for 15 to 30 minutes before and after administration of the drug, which should be given on an empty stomach. Which of the following are the possible reasons for the nurse's actions?

   a. Facilitates the drug's therapeutic action
   b. Facilitates access to the medication
   c. Facilitates mixing into the liquid form
   d. Facilitates instillation in the enteral tube

15. A nurse at the health care facility is providing the discharge instructions for an elderly client. Which of the following should the nurse include in the education regarding administration of drugs? Select all that apply.

   a. Visual description of the drug, and action, dose, and time of administration
   b. List of health care facilities where the client can receive treatment
   c. Instruction regarding whether food or liquid should accompany administration
   d. Telephone number for the health care provider to contact should side effects occur
   e. Client's insurance number should the client require emergency treatment

Topical and Inhalant Medications

SECTION I: LEARNING OBJECTIVES

- Explain how topical medications are administered.
- Give at least five examples of where topical medications are commonly applied.
- Give three examples of an inunction.
- Name two forms of drugs applied by the transdermal route.
- Discuss at least two principles nurses follow when applying a skin patch.
- Describe where eye medications are applied.
- Explain how the administration of ear medications differs for adults and children.
- Explain the rebound effect that accompanies the administration of nasal decongestants.
- Describe the difference between sublingual and buccal administration.
- Name a common reason for vaginal applications.
- Give the form of medication used most often for rectal administration.
- Explain why inhalation is a good route for medication administration.
- Describe the mechanism for creating an aerosol.
- Name two types of inhalers.
- Name a device that can maximize absorption of an inhaled medication.

SECTION II: ASSESSING YOUR UNDERSTANDING

Activity A *Fill in the blanks.*

1. A(n) _____ is a medication incorporated into an agent that is administered by rubbing it into the skin.

2. Drugs incorporated into patches or pastes are administered as _____ applications.

3. A(n) _____ contains a drug within a thick base and is applied, but not rubbed, into the skin.

4. Monitoring heart rate and blood pressure of older adults who use inhaled _____ is important because these medications commonly cause tachycardia and hypertension.

5. A(n) _____ application is a drug instilled in the outer ear.

6. A tablet given by _____ application is placed under the tongue to dissolve slowly and become absorbed by the rich blood supply in the area.

7. Symptoms of a(n) _____ infection include intense vaginal itching and a white, cheeselike vaginal discharge.

8. The _____ route administers drugs to the lower airways.

9. A(n) _____ results after a liquid drug is forced through a narrow channel using pressurized air or an inert gas.

10. Drugs administered rectally are usually in the form of _____; however, creams and ointments also may be prescribed.

Activity B *Consider the following figure.*

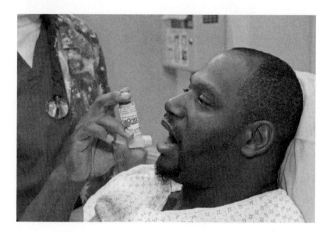

1. Identify the figure.

_____

_____

_____

2. What does the device consist of?

_____

_____

_____

Activity C *Match the terms related to topical and inhalant medications in column A with their descriptions in column B.*

Column A

_____ 1. Topical route

_____ 2. Cutaneous applications

_____ 3. Skin patches

Column B

A. Drugs rubbed into or placed in contact with the skin

B. Swelling of the nasal mucosa within a short time of drug administration

C. Drugs placed against the mucous membranes of the inner cheek

_____ 4. Rebound effect

_____ 5. Buccal application

D. Drugs bonded to an adhesive bandage and applied to the skin

E. Administration of the medication to the skin and mucous membrane

Activity D *Presented here, in random order, are steps that occur during instillation of ear medication. Write the correct sequence in the boxes provided.*

1. Instill in the opposite ear if bilateral administration is prescribed.

2. Tilt the client's head to instill prescribed drops of medication.

3. Place a small cotton ball to absorb the excess solution.

4. Manipulate the client's ear by straightening the auditory canal.

5. Instruct the client to remain in this position until the solution reaches the eardrum.

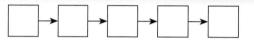

Activity E *Briefly answer the following.*

1. What are skin patches?

_____

_____

_____

2. What are otic applications?

_____

_____

_____

3. What warning should a nurse give to a client who uses over-the-counter decongestant nasal sprays frequently?

_____

_____

_____

4. What nursing instruction should a nurse give during the administration of sublingual or buccal application?

_____

_____

_____

5. What are the advantages of administering drugs through the inhalant route?

_____

_____

_____

6. What are the types of inhalers available to administer medication?

_____

_____

_____

Activity F *Use the clues to complete the crossword puzzle.*

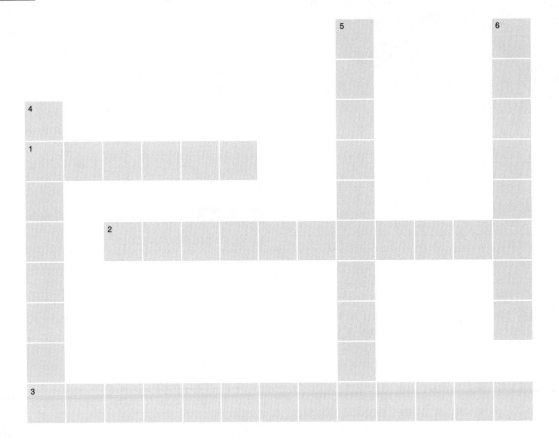

Across

1. Provides a reservoir for the aerosol medication
2. Used to relieve motion sickness
3. Used to dilate the coronary arteries

Down

4. Hormone used to treat menopausal symptoms
5. Medications supplied either in liquid form and instilled as drops or as ointments applied along the lower lid margin
6. Hand-held devices for delivering medication into the respiratory passages

SECTION III: APPLYING YOUR KNOWLEDGE

Activity G *Ophthalmic application is a method of applying drugs to the mucous membrane of one or both eyes. Answer the following question related to the nurse's role when administering ophthalmic drugs.*

A nurse is caring for a client with conjunctivitis at the health care facility.

1. What care should the nurse take when administering ophthalmic medication to this client?

_____

_____

_____

SECTION IV: PRACTICING FOR NCLEX

Activity H *Answer the following questions.*

1. A client has been ordered hydrocortisone. Which of the following nursing interventions should the nurse perform for this client when applying this inunction?
   a. Clean the area with soap and water
   b. Apply the inunction with the palm
   c. Cool the inunction before application
   d. Lightly spread the inunction over the area

2. A client has been prescribed a vaginal application for yeast infection. Which of the following should the nurse inform the client regarding administration of the vaginal application?
   a. Instill the medication in the morning after a bath
   b. Avoid emptying the bladder after application
   c. Lubricate the applicator tip with water-soluble jelly
   d. Remain recumbent for 5 minutes after application

3. A client at the health care facility has been prescribed nitroglycerin cream to dilate the coronary arteries. Which of the following routes should the nurse select to administer this medication to the client?
   a. Cutaneous
   b. Sublingual
   c. Otic
   d. Buccal

4. A client with pulmonary edema has been prescribed nitroglycerin. Which of the following is true for a drug that is described as a paste?
   a. It is bonded to an adhesive and applied to the skin
   b. It is placed against the mucous membrane of the inner cheek
   c. It is applied, but not rubbed, into the skin
   d. It is placed under the tongue and left to dissolve slowly

5. A physician prescribes the use of a contraceptive patch to a female client at the health care facility. The nurse knows that which of the following statements is true for a patch?
   a. A patch is mostly applied to the upper part of the body
   b. The drug in the patch becomes inactive immediately when the patch is removed
   c. A new patch is placed in exactly the same location as the previous one
   d. The drug in the patch takes 15 minutes to reach the therapeutic level after application

6. A nurse applies nitroglycerin paste to a client per the direction of the physician. What care should the nurse take to avoid irritating the client's skin?
   a. Avoid using the bare fingers to apply the paste
   b. Tape all edges of the application paper to the skin
   c. Remove one application before applying another
   d. Rotate the application site of the medicine

7. A nurse is caring for a client who has developed a stye in the left eye. When administering the eye medication, what should the nurse do to prevent the drug from passing into the nasolacrimal duct?

   a. Position the sleeping client with the head tilted back

   b. Instruct the client to look toward the ceiling

   c. Make a pouch in the lower lid by pulling the skin downward

   d. Instruct the client to close the eyelids gently

8. A nurse needs to monitor the heart rate and blood pressure in a client who has been prescribed the use of bronchodilators. The nurse should be aware that these medications commonly cause which of the following conditions?

   a. Bradycardia

   b. Hypertension

   c. Bronchitis

   d. Asthma

9. A client visits the health care facility with complaints of an earache resulting from an infection. The nurse needs to perform an otic application for this client. The nurse understands that an otic application is used for which of the following purposes? Select all that apply.

   a. Moistening impacted cerumen

   b. The removal of a foreign body

   c. Treating local bacterial infection

   d. Clearing the auditory canal

   e. Treating local fungal infection

10. A nurse at the health care facility is caring for a client who complains of nasal congestion resulting from swelling of the nasal mucosa. The nurse further learns that the client has been using more than the recommended dosage of nasal medication. What should the nurse suggest to avoid this condition?

   a. Use a nasal spray that contains normal saline solution

   b. Use a nasal spray that contains a decreased dose of the medication

   c. Use a nasal spray that contains anti-inflammatory medication

   d. Use a nasal spray that contains antiallergy medication

11. A client has been prescribed nasal drops for difficulty in breathing resulting from severe nasal congestion. What should the nurse do to distribute the medication?

   a. Place a rolled towel or pillow behind the client's neck

   b. Instruct the client to breathe as the container is squeezed

   c. Aim the tip of the dropper toward the nasal passage

   d. Instruct the client to breathe through the mouth

12. The physician has prescribed sublingual application of medication for a client with hypertension. Which of the following should the nurse tell the client is the right method of administration of the drug?

   a. Place the drug against the mucous membrane of the inner cheek

   b. Administer the drug by rubbing it into the skin

   c. Place the drug under the tongue and allow it to dissolve slowly

   d. Place the adhesive bandage, which is bonded to the drug, onto the skin

13. A nurse at the health care facility needs to administer nasal medication to a client with complaints of breathing difficulty. Before administering the medication, what should the nurse do to ensure that the right drug is given at the right time by the right route?

   a. Administer the medication 30 to 60 minutes within the scheduled time

   b. Read and compare the labels on the drug with the MAR

   c. Compare the MAR with the written medical record

   d. Review the client's drug, allergy, and medical histories

14. A client visits the health care facility for a routine physical assessment. During the assessment, the client complains to the nurse that recently she has been experiencing intense itching around the vaginal area and has noticed a white, cheeselike discharge. The nurse is aware that these are symptoms of a yeast infection. The nurse should be aware that which of the following medications would help to relieve the client's condition?

a. Suppository cream

b. Scopolamine

c. Nitroglycerin cream

d. Estrogen

15. An asthmatic client has been prescribed the use of a turbo inhaler. The nurse understands that which of the following describes the mechanism of a turbo inhaler?

a. A device that forces a liquid drug through a narrow channel using pressurized air

b. A device that consists of a canister that releases a dose of medication when compressed

c. A device that forces medication with the help of inert gas through a narrow channel

d. A propeller-driven device that spins and suspends a finely powdered medication

34

Parenteral Medications

SECTION I: LEARNING OBJECTIVES

- Name three parts of a syringe.
- List five factors to consider when selecting a syringe and needle.
- Explain the rationale for redesigning conventional syringes and needles.
- Name three ways that pharmaceutical companies prepare parenteral drugs.
- Discuss an appropriate action before combining two drugs in a single syringe.
- List four injection routes.
- Identify common sites for intradermal, subcutaneous, and intramuscular injections.
- Name a type of syringe commonly used to administer an intradermal, subcutaneous, and intramuscular injection.
- Describe the angles of entry for intradermal, subcutaneous, and intramuscular injections.
- Discuss why most insulin combinations must be administered within 15 minutes of being mixed.
- Describe two techniques for preventing bruising when administering heparin subcutaneously.

SECTION II: ASSESSING YOUR UNDERSTANDING

Activity A *Fill in the blanks.*

1. The dorsogluteal site should be avoided when administering an intramuscular injection because of the risk of damaging the _____ nerve.

2. Nurses draw an imaginary line at the _____ when administering an injection in the deltoid site.

3. A(n) _____ syringe holds 1 mL fluid and is calibrated in 0.01-mL increments.

4. When administering _____ injections, nurses use a 90-degree angle for piercing the skin.

5. _____ is unnecessary when injecting insulin with an insulin pen.

6. There is a risk of damaging the _____ nerve and artery if the deltoid site is not identified properly.

7. _____ syringes and needles are being redesigned to avoid needle-stick injuries.

8. _____ is the process of adding a diluent to a powdered substance before administering the drug parenterally.

9. _____ needles provide a barrier for glass particles when withdrawing medication from a glass ampule.

10. _____ is a hormone required by some clients with diabetes.

Activity B *Consider the following figures.*

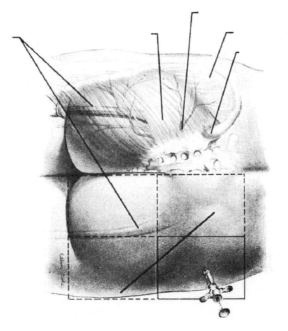

1. Identify and label the image.

   _____

   _____

   _____

2. Which is the primary muscle in this injection site?

   _____

   _____

   _____

3. Identify the method shown in the image.

   _____

   _____

   _____

4. Why is this method performed?

   _____

   _____

   _____

Activity C *Match the type of injection in column A with the size of syringe used in column B.*

Column A

____ **1.** Intradermal

____ **2.** Subcutaneous

____ **3.** Insulin

____ **4.** Intramuscular

Column B

A. 3 or 5 mL calibrated in 0.2-mL increments

B. 1 mL calibrated in units

C. 1, 2, 2.5, or 3 mL calibrated in 0.1-mL increments

D. 1 mL calibrated in 0.01 mL in minims

Activity D *Presented here, in random order, are steps that occur during the withdrawal of medication from an ampule. Write the correct sequence in the boxes provided.*

1. Tap the top of the ampule.

2. Tap the barrel of the syringe near the hub.

3. Insert the needle into the ampule.

4. Snap the neck of the ampule.

5. Remove the filter needle and attach a sterile needle.

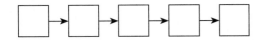

Activity E *Briefly answer the following.*

1. What is the meaning of parenteral route?

_____

_____

_____

2. What are the components of a syringe?

_____

_____

_____

3. Why is a lower drug dose indicated in elderly clients?

_____

_____

_____

4. Why is it important to pinch tissue for an intramuscular injection?

_____

_____

_____

5. Why are conventional syringes and needles being redesigned?

_____

_____

_____

6. Why is it important to rotate insulin injection sites?

_____

_____

_____

Activity F *Use the clues to complete the crossword puzzle.*

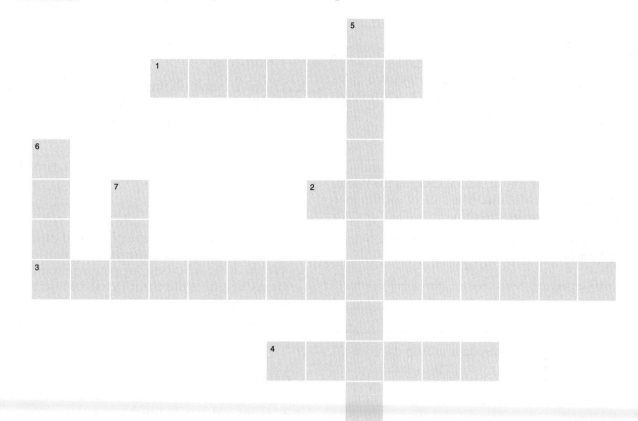

Across

1. It contains 50/50 amounts of intermediate-acting and short-acting insulins
2. It is the part of the syringe that holds the medication
3. Buildup of subcutaneous fat at the site of repeated insulin injection
4. A sealed glass drug container broken to withdraw the medication

Down

5. Breakdown of subcutaneous fat at the site of repeated insulin injections
6. A glass container of parenteral medication with a self-sealing rubber stopper
7. The part of the syringe to which the needle is attached

SECTION III: APPLYING YOUR KNOWLEDGE

Activity G *The most common route for administering insulin is through a subcutaneous or intravenous injection. However, an inhaled form of insulin called Exubera has recently been approved. Answer the following questions, which involve the nurse's role in caring for a diabetic client.*

A nurse is caring for a client who is obese and has diabetes. The physician has ordered the nurse to administer a combined low dose of insulin to the client per the prescription.

1. What type of syringe should the nurse use to administer the insulin?

_____

_____

_____

2. When should the nurse administer the combined low dose of insulin to the client?

_____

_____

_____

SECTION IV: PRACTICING FOR NCLEX

Activity H *Answer the following questions.*

1. A nurse has reconstituted a prescribed vial drug for administering to a client. Which of the following actions should the nurse perform if the medication needs to be reused for more than one administration?
   a. Write the client's name on the vial label
   b. Write the date, time, and initials on the vial label
   c. Write the client's illness on the vial label
   d. Write the syringe details on the vial label

2. A nurse needs to administer an intramuscular injection to a client in the rectus femoris site. Which of the following actions should the nurse perform? Select all that apply.
   a. Palpate the posterior iliac spine and greater trochanter
   b. Place the injection in the middle third of the thigh
   c. Ask the client to lie in a supine position on the bed
   d. Ask the client to sit on the edge of the bed
   e. Place one hand on the knee and below the trochanter

3. A nurse is administering a heparin injection subcutaneously to a client. What is the normal gauge of a needle when administering medications subcutaneously?
   a. 25 gauge
   b. 27 gauge
   c. 20 gauge
   d. 23 gauge

4. A nurse has administered a prescribed injection to a client in the dorsogluteal site. Which of the following suggestions should the nurse give to the client to reduce injection discomfort?
   a. Massage the injection with local anesthetic
   b. Take deep breaths before receiving the injection
   c. Lie in a prone position and point the toes outward
   d. Avoid ambulating for 10 minutes after receiving the injection

5. A nurse is withdrawing medication from an ampule. Which of the following techniques should the nurse follow to prevent injecting glass particles into the client?
   a. Insert the filter needle into the ampule
   b. Tap the barrel of the syringe near the hub
   c. Use a needle with a small diameter
   d. Attach a sterile needle for administering the injection

6. Per the physician's order, a nurse is combining two prescribed drugs into a single syringe. Which of the following actions should the nurse perform before combining the two drugs?
   a. Use a larger gauge needle for combining drugs
   b. Withdraw an equal amount of drug from their containers
   c. Consult a drug reference chart before withdrawing
   d. Fix a filter needle on the syringe before withdrawing

7. A nurse is withdrawing a prescribed narcotic drug from a vial to administer it to a client with chronic back pain. Which of the following measures should the nurse take to prevent illegal drug use of the excess medication?

   a. Avoid discarding the excess medication in the trash

   b. Label the vial container with a secret code

   c. Aspirate and dispose of the excess medication in the presence of a witness

   d. Dilute the excess medication with saline solution

8. A nurse needs to administer an intramuscular injection to a client. Which of the following ways can the nurse reduce injection discomfort?

   a. Avoid changing needles when there is tissue irritation

   b. Apply an ice pack to numb the skin before the injection

   c. Avoid applying pressure to the site when removing the needle

   d. Instill the medication quickly and steadily

9. A nurse needs to flush all the medication from the syringe at the time of injection. Which of the following actions should the nurse perform?

   a. Use a needle with a smaller gauge

   b. Attach a long shaft needle to the syringe

   c. Avoid using filter needles when withdrawing

   d. Add 0.1 to 0.2 mL air to the syringe

10. A nurse is assessing the stock of safety injection devices in the health care facility. Which of the following are modified safety injection devices? Select all that apply.

    a. Injections with plastic shields that cover the needle after use

    b. Injections with reusable needles that are immersed in an alcohol solution

    c. Injections with disposable needles that are cleaned with cotton swabs

    d. Injections with needles that retract into the syringe

    e. Gas-pressured devices that inject medications without needles

11. A nurse has placed one hand above the knee and one hand below the greater trochanter of a client before administering a prescribed intramuscular injection to an infant. Which of the following sites is the nurse administering the injection?

    a. Deltoid site

    b. Vastus lateralis site

    c. Rectus femoris site

    d. Ventrogluteal site

12. A nurse has administered a prescribed dosage of heparin injection to a client subcutaneously. Which of the following actions should the nurse remember to perform when administering a heparin injection?

    a. Administer the dosages of heparin in small volumes

    b. Use the same needle for withdrawing and administering heparin

    c. Avoid rotating injection sites when administering heparin

    d. Massage the injection site after administering injection

13. A nurse is bunching the tissue of a client between the thumb and fingers before administering an injection to the client subcutaneously. The nurse knows that which of the following clients are preferred for the bunching technique? Select all that apply.

    a. Diabetic clients

    b. Infants

    c. Children

    d. Thin clients

    e. Obese clients

14. A nurse needs to administer an irritating medication to a client. Which of the following injections is most suitable for an irritating medication?

    a. Intravenous

    b. Subcutaneous

    c. Intradermal

    d. Intramuscular

15. A nurse is administering an intramuscular injection to a client in the ventrogluteal site. What are the advantages offered by this site over the dorsogluteal site?

   a. It has large nerves and blood vessels

   b. It is less fatty and fecal contamination is rare

   c. It can hold a large amount of injected medication

   d. It can be massaged immediately after injection

16. A nurse is mixing insulins before administering them to a client with diabetes. Which of the following actions should the nurse perform to mix the insulins without damaging the protein molecules?

   a. Administer it within 15 minutes of mixing

   b. Insert the needle in the insulin itself

   c. Roll the medication in the palms

   d. Withdraw specific units of insulin from the vial with an additive

Intravenous Medications

SECTION I: LEARNING OBJECTIVES

- Name two types of veins into which intravenous medications are administered.
- Describe at least three appropriate situations for administering intravenous medications.
- Name two ways intravenous medications are administered.
- Describe one method for giving bolus administrations of intravenous medications.
- Describe two methods for administering medicated solutions intermittently.
- Explain the technique for administering a piggyback infusion.
- Discuss two purposes for using a volume-control set.
- Describe a central venous catheter.
- Name three types of central venous catheters.
- Discuss two techniques for protecting oneself when administering antineoplastic drugs.

SECTION II: ASSESSING YOUR UNDERSTANDING

Activity A *Fill in the blanks.*

1. Nurses pour 70% of _____ over any antineoplastic drug spill to inactivate the drug.

2. Elderly clients with _____ often experience more confusion and disorientation with an acute illness.

3. A(n) _____ catheter is inserted through the skin in a peripheral vein such as the jugular or subclavian vein.

4. A(n) _____ administration is also described as a drug given by intravenous push.

5. The _____ attaches a special label to a container of antineoplastic drugs to warn nurses.

6. The end of the tunnel catheter exits from the skin lateral to the _____ process.

7. A(n) _____ lock is also called a *saline* or *heparin lock,* or an *intermittent infusion device.*

8. _____ drugs are commonly also referred to as *chemotherapy* or just *chemo.*

9. Most _____ catheters are inserted by a physician and then sutured to the skin.

10. _____ catheters have a self-sealing port pierced through the skin with a special needle.

Activity B *Consider the following figures.*

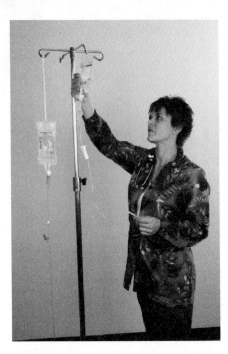

1. Identify the image.

_____

_____

_____

2. What is the advantage of this arrangement?

_____

_____

_____

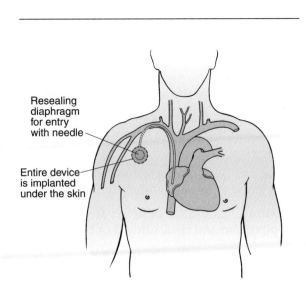

Resealing diaphragm for entry with needle

Entire device is implanted under the skin

3. Identify the image.

_____

_____

_____

4. What is the advantage of this arrangement?

_____

_____

_____

Activity C *Match the types of intravenous administration in column A with their features in column B.*

Column A

____ **1.** Bolus administration

____ **2.** Continuous administration

____ **3.** Secondary infusion

____ **4.** Volume-control set

Column B

A. Parenteral drug that is instilled over several hours

B. Intravenous tubing chamber that holds a portion of the solution

C. Undiluted medication given quickly into a vein

D. Parenteral drug that has been diluted in a small volume of intravenous solution

Activity D *Presented here, in random order, are steps that occur during administration of medication through an intravenous port. Write the correct sequence in the boxes provided.*

1. Pull back the plunger of the syringe.

2. Gently instill a few tenths of a milliliter of medication.

3. Locate the port nearest to the intravenous insertion site.

4. Pierce the port with needle and pinch the tubing.

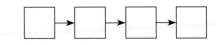

Activity E *Briefly answer the following.*

1. When is it appropriate to seek another drug route for elderly clients?

_____

_____

_____

2. How is a bolus administration given to a client?

_____

_____

_____

3. What is a medication lock?

_____

_____

_____

4. What is the purpose of antineoplastic drugs?

_____

_____

_____

5. What is a central venous catheter?

_____

_____

_____

6. What information should the nurse provide to clients about intravenous route drugs?

_____

_____

_____

Activity F *Use the clues to complete the crossword puzzle.*

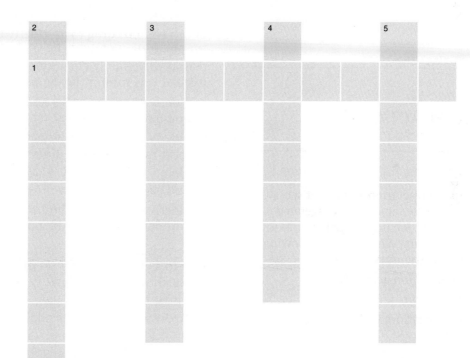

Across

1. A route of drug administration that provides an immediate effect

Down

2. Another name used for secondary infusion
3. A commonly used tunneled catheter
4. A solution used to maintain the patency of implanted catheters
5. A commercial name for a volume-control set

SECTION III: APPLYING YOUR KNOWLEDGE

Activity G *Elderly clients comprise the largest age group of clients cared for in acute and long-term health care facilities. Administration of intravenous medications is quite common in elderly clients. Answer the following questions, which involve the nurse's role in caring for clients on intravenous therapy.*

A nurse is preparing the discharge sheet of an elderly client with an intravenous drug administered to him through a tunneled catheter.

1. What should the nurse do if the client needs continued intravenous therapy?

   _____

   _____

   _____

2. What should a nurse teach to an elderly client when there is emphasis on an early discharge?

   _____

   _____

   _____

SECTION IV: PRACTICING FOR NCLEX

Activity H *Answer the following questions.*

1. When administering an intermittent secondary infusion, a nurse removes a refrigerated secondary solution 30 minutes before administering it to the client. Which of the following reasons explains the nurse's action?
   a. Ensures medication accuracy
   b. Promotes comfort
   c. Prevents medication errors
   d. Ensures client safety

2. A nurse is administering antineoplastic drugs to a client with cancer. Which are the possible ways through which nurses or caregivers can absorb antineoplastic drugs? Select all that apply.
   a. Through skin contact
   b. Through inhalation of fluid droplets
   c. Through oral intake of drug residue
   d. Through radiation of heat
   e. Through chemical vapors

3. A nurse is administering intravenous medication to a client with the aid of a medication lock. Which of the following is the most popular feature of a medication lock?
   a. It eliminates the need for a continuous administration of intravenous fluid
   b. It can be flushed with saline and heparin
   c. It can withstand approximately 2,000 punctures
   d. It can maintain patency without obtaining a blood return

4. A nurse is administering a prescribed dosage of intravenous drug to an elderly client. Which of the following factors explain the reason why elderly clients are predisposed to toxic effects from intravenous drugs?
   a. Elderly clients have decreased visual acuity and manual dexterity
   b. Elderly clients face confusion and disorientation with an acute illness
   c. Elderly clients have a slower metabolism and excretion process
   d. Elderly clients have diminished protein components in their blood

5. A nurse is administering intravenous medication to a client with the aid of a Soluset. The nurse knows that a Soluset is used for which of the following functions?
   a. To ensure the need for additional intravenous fluid
   b. To administer parenteral medication in a large volume of blood
   c. To stabilize catheters and reduce the potential for infection
   d. To avoid overloading the circulatory system

6. A nurse needs to use a central venous catheter to administer 150 mL medication to a client. Which of the following steps should the nurse perform to prevent complications such as air embolism?

   a. Regulate the flow of infusion
   b. Reclamp the catheter
   c. Remove the needle from the port
   d. Instill 5 mL normal saline in tubing

7. A nurse is caring for an elderly client who is being administered an intravenous drug intermittently. The nurse knows that he or she should observe elderly clients for adverse effects of which of the following drugs? Select all that apply.

   a. Anticoagulants
   b. Opiates
   c. Insulin
   d. Sulfonamides
   e. Normal saline

8. A nurse opens the lower clamp of a volume-control set until it is filled with fluid and then clamps it before administering a prescribed intravenous drug to a client. Which of the following reasons explains the nurse's action?

   a. To fill the drip chamber with fluid
   b. To prepare the equipment for administration
   c. To permit fluid to enter the calibrated container
   d. To purge unwanted air from the tubing

9. A nurse is assessing the condition of a client with an implanted catheter. The client complains of skin discomfort to the nurse. Which of the following actions should the nurse perform to reduce the skin discomfort?

   a. Replace the special needle
   b. Apply anesthetic topically
   c. Change the self-sealing port
   d. Cease the intravenous solution

10. A nurse needs to dilute a parenteral drug in a secondary infusion before delivering the prescribed dosage to the client. What is the volume of intravenous solution that is usually used to dilute during a second infusion?

    a. 100 to 250 mL over 5 to 60 minutes
    b. 500 to 1,000 mL over 5 to 6 hours
    c. 100 to 500 mL over 30 to 60 minutes
    d. 50 to 100 mL over 30 to 60 minutes

11. A nurse is assessing the health of a client who has a prescribed dosage of bolus administration after a cesarean operation. The client is showing symptoms of accidental hypothermia. Which of the following actions should the nurse perform when a client's condition changes for any reason during a bolus administration?

    a. Call for the lead physician
    b. Stop the administration of intravenous fluid
    c. Reduce the prescribed rate of intravenous fluid
    d. Call the emergency service for help

12. When preparing a prescribed dosage of an antineoplastic drug, the nurse covers the drug preparation area with a disposable paper pad. Which of the following reasons explain the nurse's action?

    a. To reduce the potential of skin contact
    b. To inactivate the prescribed drug
    c. To avoid inhalation of the drug spill
    d. To absorb a small drug spill

13. A nurse needs to administer an intravenous medication to a client through an intermittent infusion device. Which of the following solutions is used to fill the intravenous tubing before administration?

    a. Sterile bacteriostatic water
    b. Sterile normal water
    c. Sterile isopropyl alcohol
    d. Sterile hydrogen peroxide

14. A nurse is administering intravenous medications and fluid to an elderly client. The client complains to the nurse about a bloated abdomen and frequent urination. The nurse stops the intravenous administration and fixes the volume-control set to administer the intravenous medications and fluids. Which of the following nursing diagnoses should the nurse identify?

a. Risk for injury

b. Risk for infection

c. Excess fluid volume

d. Acute pain

15. A nurse is administering an intermittent secondary infusion to a client. Which of the following actions does the nurse perform when administering an intermittent secondary infusion? Select all that apply.

a. Hang the secondary solution higher than the primary solution

b. Avoid inserting the modified adapter within the port

c. Avoid clamping the tubing when the solution has instilled

d. Release the roller clamp on the secondary solution

e. Regulate the rate of flow by counting the drip rate

CHAPTER 36

Airway Management

SECTION I: LEARNING OBJECTIVES

■ Define airway management.
■ Identify the structural components of the airway.
■ Discuss four natural mechanisms that protect the airway.
■ Explain methods nurses use to help maintain the natural airway.
■ Name two techniques for liquefying respiratory secretions.
■ Explain the three techniques of chest physiotherapy.
■ Describe at least three suctioning techniques used to clear secretions from the airway.
■ Discuss two indications for inserting an artificial airway.
■ Name two examples of artificial airways.
■ Identify three components of tracheostomy care.

SECTION II: ASSESSING YOUR UNDERSTANDING

Activity A *Fill in the blanks.*

1. The _____ is a protrusion of flexible cartilage above the larynx.

2. Hairlike projections called _____ beat debris upward that collects in the lower airway.

3. The volume of water in mucus affects its _____, or thickness.

4. _____ therapy improves breathing, encourages spontaneous coughing, and helps clients to raise sputum for diagnostic purposes.

5. Evaluation of _____ is important for implementing appropriate interventions to prevent aspiration.

6. _____ relies on negative pressure to remove liquid secretions with a catheter.

7. Nurses perform _____ suctioning with a suctioning device called a Yankeur-tip or tonsil-tip catheter.

8. _____ suctioning means removing secretions from the upper portion of the lower airway through a nasally inserted catheter.

9. A nasopharyngeal airway, sometimes called a(n) _____ can be used to protect the nostril if frequent suctioning is necessary.

10. Respiratory cilia become less efficient with age, predisposing older adults to a high incidence of _____.

Activity B *Consider the following figures.*

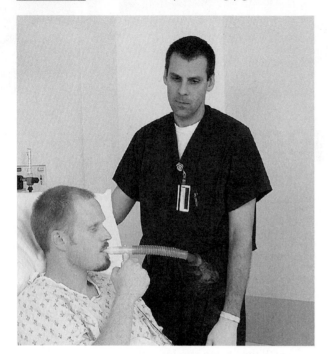

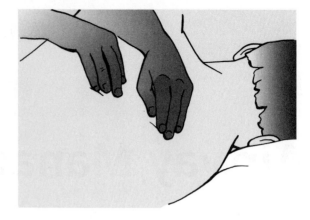

3. Identify the type of postural drainage technique used here.

_____

_____

_____

4. What is the purpose of this technique?

_____

_____

_____

1. Identify the type of therapy being performed here.

_____

_____

_____

2. How does this therapy help the client?

_____

_____

_____

Activity C *Match each term related to airway management in column A with its description in column B.*

Column A

___ **1.** Ventilation

___ **2.** Inhalation therapy

___ **3.** Chest physiotherapy

___ **4.** Postural drainage

___ **5.** Oropharyngeal suctioning

Column B

A. Respiratory treatments that provide a mixture of oxygen, humidification, and aerosolized medications directly to the lungs

B. Positioning technique that promotes gravity drainage of secretions from various lobes or segments of the lungs

C. Removing secretions from the throat through an orally inserted catheter

D. Indicated for clients with chronic respiratory diseases who have difficulty coughing or raising thick mucus

E. Movement of air in and out of the lung

Activity D *Presented here, in random order, are the steps that occur when the nurse performs percussion on a client. Write the correct sequence in the boxes provided.*

1. Keep the fingers and thumb together.

2. Percuss for 3 to 5 minutes in each postural drainage position.

3. Cup the hands.

4. Apply the cupped hands to the client's chest.

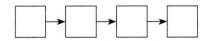

Activity E *Briefly answer the following.*

1. What are the factors that can jeopardize airway patency?

_____

_____

_____

2. What are the structures that protect the airway from a wide variety of inhaled substances?

_____

_____

_____

3. What are the most common methods of maintaining the natural airway?

_____

_____

_____

4. What are the two common types of artificial airway management?

_____

_____

_____

5. What is the purpose of an oral airway?

_____

_____

_____

6. What are the common causes of pathologic pulmonary changes in elderly clients?

_____

_____

_____

Activity F *Use the clues to complete the crossword puzzle.*

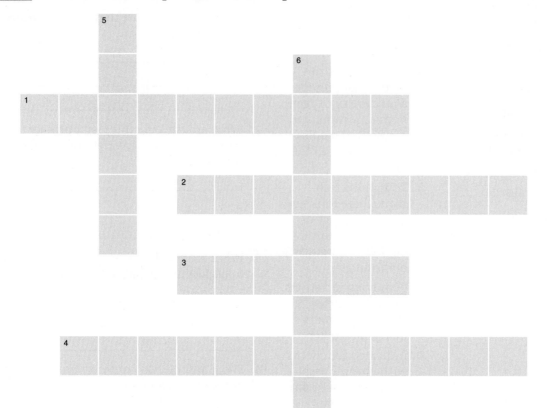

Across

1. Helps to dislodge respiratory secretions that adhere to the bronchial walls
2. Process of providing adequate fluid intake to keep mucous membranes moist and mucus thin
3. Mucus raised to the level of the upper airways
4. A surgically created opening into the trachea

Down

5. The collective system of tubes in the upper and lower respiratory tract
6. The process of using the palms of the hands to shake underlying tissue and loosen retained secretions

SECTION III: APPLYING YOUR KNOWLEDGE

Activity G *Clients at risk for airway obstruction or requiring long-term mechanical ventilation are candidates for an artificial airway. Answer the following question related to the nursing care for a client with a tracheostomy tube.*

A nurse is caring for a client who requires prolonged mechanical ventilation and oxygenation.

1. What intervention should the nurse perform for the client who is unable to talk because of the tracheostomy tube?

   _____

   _____

   _____

SECTION IV: PRACTICING FOR NCLEX

Activity H *Answer the following questions.*

1. The nurse is caring for an asthmatic client at the health care facility. The nurse is aware that which of the following structures form part of the lower airway? Select all that apply.
   a. Trachea
   b. Nose
   c. Bronchi
   d. Alveoli
   e. Pharynx

2. A client at the health care facility is being treated for an injury to the tracheal cartilages. The nurse understands that which of the following statements is the function of the tracheal cartilages?
   a. Act as a lid that closes during swallowing and help direct food
   b. Ensure a portion of the airway beneath the larynx remains open
   c. Type of tissue that lines the respiratory passage to trap particulate matter
   d. Hairlike projections that beat debris collected in lower airways

3. A nurse uses aerosol therapy for a client with complaints of chest congestion. The nurse is aware that which of the following is the benefit of aerosol therapy?
   a. Helps in raising sputum for diagnostic purposes
   b. Helps in dislodging respiratory secretions
   c. Helps in loosening retained secretions
   d. Helps in draining secretions from various lobes of the lungs

4. A nurse at the health care facility needs to send a client's sputum specimen to the laboratory for diagnostic purposes. Which of the following timing allows the collection of a specimen when more mucous is available?
   a. Just before the client goes to sleep
   b. Just after the client undergoes physiotherapy

   c. Just after the client awakens
   d. Just after percussion is performed on the client

5. A client with a chronic respiratory disorder has been prescribed a postural drainage technique by the physician. The nurse understands that which of the following is the outcome of postural drainage?
   a. Promotes gravity drainage of secretion
   b. Encourages spontaneous coughing
   c. Helps loosen retained secretions
   d. Helps dislodge respiratory secretions

6. A physician directs the nurse to perform percussion on a client who is having difficulty coughing. During therapy, how long should the nurse perform percussion on each postural drainage position?
   a. For 3 to 5 minutes
   b. For 10 minutes
   c. For 10 to 15 minutes
   d. For 15 minutes

7. A nurse is caring for an infant client with chest congestion. The doctor has ordered the nurse to use suctioning to relieve the client's condition. What negative pressure should be applied for the infant if the nurse uses a wall suctioning machine?
   a. 100 to 140 mm Hg
   b. 50 to 85 mm Hg
   c. 95 to 100 mm Hg
   d. 45 to 50 mm Hg

8. A nurse has been directed to use suction to relieve a client with chest congestion. When performing the suctioning, what should the nurse do to break up mucus and raise secretions?
   a. Occlude the air vent of the suction
   b. Rotate the catheter, as it is withdrawn
   c. Encourage the client to cough
   d. Wait until the client takes a breath

9. A physician directs the nurse to use nasopharyngeal suctioning for a client with chest congestion. The nurse should be aware that which of the following describes nasopharyngeal suctioning?

   a. Removing secretions from the throat through a nasally inserted catheter

   b. Removing secretions from the upper portion of the lower airway through a nasally inserted catheter

   c. Removing secretions from the throat through an orally inserted catheter

   d. Removing secretions from the mouth using a Yankeur-tip or tonsil-tip catheter

10. When caring for clients who require an artificial airway at the health care facility, the nurse should understand that which of the following clients are candidates for a tracheostomy? Select all that apply.

    a. A client recovering from general anesthesia

    b. A client who has an upper airway obstruction

    c. A client recovering from a seizure

    d. A client who requires prolonged mechanical ventilation

    e. A client who is less stable and requires oxygenation

11. A nurse is caring for a client who is recovering from surgery for removal of a brain tumor. The nurse uses an oral airway to manage the client's airway. What should the nurse do to prevent aspiration in the client?

    a. Perform oral suctioning if necessary

    b. Position the client supine with the neck hyperextended

    c. Hold the airway so that the curved tip points upward

    d. Rotate the airway over the top of the tongue

12. A client at the health care facility is receiving mechanical ventilation through a tracheostomy tube. The nurse needs to perform suctioning because of the presence of copious secretions. The nurse inserts the catheter tube a shorter distance—that is, until resistance is felt. The nurse should understand that which of the following is the possible cause of resistance?

    a. Contact between the catheter tip and the main bronchi

    b. Contact between the carina and the main bronchi

    c. Contact between the catheter tip and the carina

    d. Contact between the catheter tip and the end of the tube

13. A nurse needs to perform tracheostomy care for a client on mechanical ventilation. Which of the following interventions should the nurse perform for tracheostomy care? Select all that apply.

    a. Cleaning the skin around the stoma

    b. Changing the outer cannula

    c. Changing the inner dressing

    d. Clearing the outer airway

    e. Cleaning the inner cannula

14. A nurse is caring for an elderly client with pneumonia. The nurse should be aware that which of the following age-related changes predisposes elderly clients to a higher incidence of pneumonia?

    a. Retention of secretions

    b. Diminished efficiency of cilia

    c. Decreased air exchange

    d. Compromised ventilation

15. The nurse is caring for an elderly client who complains of difficulty in coughing. What intervention should the nurse perform for this client? Select all that apply.

    a. Inquire about the client's current history of cough

    b. Determine how long the cough has been present

    c. Inquire whether the physician has been informed

    d. Observe and describe sputum if present

    e. Check the client's medication against the medical order

16. The nurse at the health care facility is caring for a client with difficulty swallowing (or dysphagia). The nurse should be aware that clients with dysphagia are vulnerable to which of the following conditions?

    a. Cardiac dysrhythmias

    b. Hypoxemia

    c. Aspiration pneumonia

    d. Chronic pulmonary diseases

Resuscitation

SECTION I: LEARNING OBJECTIVES

- Explain why an airway obstruction is life threatening.
- Give at least three signs of an airway obstruction.
- Describe two appropriate actions if a client has a partial airway obstruction.
- Explain the purpose of the Heimlich maneuver.
- Describe the circumstances for using subdiaphragmatic thrusts and chest thrusts.
- Discuss the technique used to dislodge an object from an infant's airway.
- Identify the recommended action for relieving an airway obstruction in an unconscious person.
- List the four steps in the chain of survival.
- Explain CPR and its associated "ABCs."
- Name two techniques for opening the airway.
- List three ways to administer rescue breathing.
- Describe the purpose of chest compression.
- Discuss the appropriate use of an automated external defibrillator.
- Identify the maximum time allowed for interrupting CPR.
- Name at least three criteria used in the decision to discontinue resuscitation efforts.

SECTION II: ASSESSING YOUR UNDERSTANDING

Activity A *Fill in the blanks.*

1. To open the airway of a person with cardiac arrest, nurses position the client _____ on a firm surface.

2. Nurses place a breathing client in the _____ position to maintain an open airway and prevent aspiration of fluid.

3. Giving a breath that lasts a full second reduces the potential for distending the _____ and stomach.

4. Squeezing the heart between the _____ and vertebrae increases pressure in the ventricles.

5. A(n) _____ of food or some other foreign object may cause mechanical airway obstruction.

6. When performing CPR, elderly clients are at a greater risk for fractured _____.

7. Nurses perform _____ breathing through the victim's mouth, nose, or stoma.

8. Correct placement of the _____ and the body is essential during chest compressions.

9. Unrelieved airway obstruction will lead to loss of _____ and eventually death.

10. A _____ team comprises of a group of people trained and certified in advanced cardiac life support.

Activity B *Consider the following figures.*

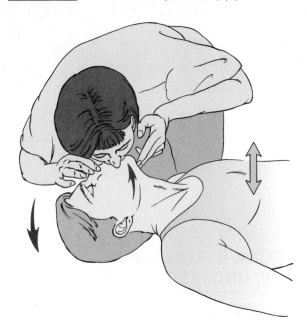

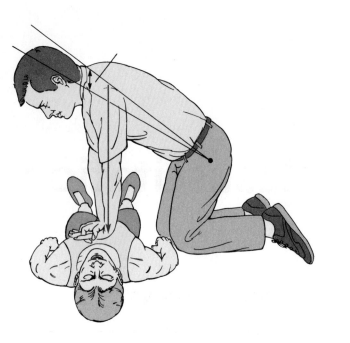

3. Identify and label the image.

_____

_____

_____

1. Identify the image.

_____

_____

_____

4. How do nurses assess whether this procedure is required?

_____

_____

_____

2. How is the action shown in the figure performed?

_____

_____

_____

Activity C *Match the different resuscitation techniques in column A with their specific features in column B.*

Column A

___ **1.** Mouth-to-mouth breathing

___ **2.** Mouth-to-nose breathing

___ **3.** Mouth-to-stoma breathing

___ **4.** Chest compression

Column B

A. Rescuer closes the infant or child's mouth

B. Promotes circulation and increases pressure in the ventricles

C. Reduces the potential for distending the esophagus

D. Rescuers use a tube with the mouth or a one-way valve mask

Activity D *Presented here, in random order, are the steps that occur during Heimlich thrusts performed on infants. Write the correct sequence in the boxes provided.*

1. Give thrusts of one per second to the middle of the breastbone just below the nipple line.

2. Use the heel of the hand to give five back slaps between the shoulder blades.

3. Turn the infant supine, and with two fingers give five chest thrusts.

4. Support the infant over the forearm and hold the infant prone with the head downward.

5. Repeatedly give five back blows and chest thrusts until the object is dislodged.

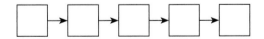

Activity E *Briefly answer the following.*

1. What is partial airway obstruction?

_____

_____

_____

2. What is rescue breathing?

_____

_____

_____

3. When is meant by the ABCDs of the cardio-pulmonary resuscitation technique?

_____

_____

_____

4. When is mouth-to-nose breathing performed?

_____

_____

_____

5. What is an automated external defibrillator (AED)?

_____

_____

_____

6. Why should a one-way mask be used when performing rescue breathing?

_____

_____

_____

Activity F *Use the clues to complete the crossword puzzle.*

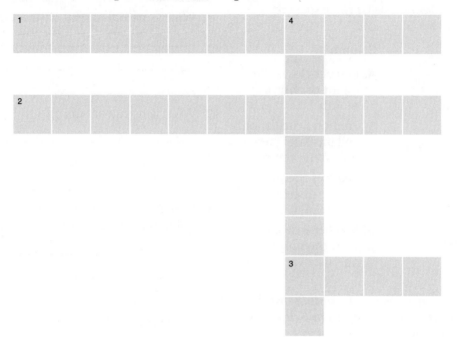

Across

1. Defective cardiac rhythm noticed in elderly clients
2. Rescuers perform CPR if the client is in this state
3. It is used to summon personnel trained in advanced life support techniques

Down

4. Common method for relieving a mechanical airway obstruction

SECTION III: APPLYING YOUR KNOWLEDGE

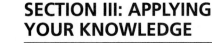 *Older adults need to be informed that they may change their minds about advance directives and instructions for resuscitation at any time. All changes must be communicated to the physician, and a written copy should be stored in a safe location. Answer the following questions, which involve the nurse's role in caring for elderly clients.*

A nurse is taking care of an elderly client who has been complaining of mild pain in the chest. The client has had two cardiac arrests in the past, and after initial assessment, the physician has ordered the nurse to keep the CPR equipment ready.

1. Why are elderly clients at a greater risk when CPR is performed on them?

   _____

   _____

   _____

2. Which type of elderly clients are more apt to bleed internally during chest compressions?

   _____

   _____

   _____

SECTION IV: PRACTICING FOR NCLEX

Activity H *Answer the following questions.*

1. A nurse needs to perform the chin lift technique on an adult client who has a partial airway obstruction. Which of the following positions is best suited for the chin lift technique?

   a. Lateral position
   b. Fowler's position
   c. Supine position
   d. Sims' position

2. A nurse is attending to a client with an airway obstruction. Which of the following evidence should the nurse notice before performing a Heimlich maneuver on the client?

   a. Insufficient chewing
   b. Compromised swallowing
   c. Inability to speak
   d. Aspiration of vomitus

3. A nurse is preparing to administer a shock with the aid of an AED to a client. Which of the following clients are not recommended for an AED shock?

   a. Clients with dementia
   b. Clients 8 years of age or younger
   c. Clients with a pacemaker
   d. Clients with osteoporosis

4. A nurse needs to administer a shock to a client with an implanted defibrillator. On which of the following places should the nurse place the AED pads?

   a. Place them on the implanted device itself
   b. Place them between the sternum and vertebrae
   c. Place them 1 inch away from implanted device
   d. Place them on the brachial artery in the upper arm

5. A nurse is performing CPR on a client without defibrillation. The nurse knows that he or she should assess the client's condition after how many cycles of compression and ventilations?

   a. Five cycles
   b. 10 cycles
   c. 15 cycles
   d. 20 cycles

6. A nurse who is part of emergency services is caring for a client who had cardiac arrest. Which of the following steps should the nurse take to initiate the chain of survival? Select all that apply.

   a. Provide the client with early CPR
   b. Arrange for the cardiac defibrillator
   c. Place the client in a recovery position
   d. Keep the advanced life support services ready
   e. Assess the client's pulse rate and circulation

7. A person accidentally swallows a large piece of food that causes partial airway obstruction. Which is the initial color on a person's face when there is partial or complete obstruction?

   a. Red
   b. Pink
   c. Blue
   d. White

8. A nurse is attaching an AED to a middle-age client who had cardiac arrest. Which of the following places have accessibility to an AED? Select all that apply.

   a. Schools

   b. Airports

   c. Police stations

   d. Amusement parks

   e. Subways

9. A nurse needs to assess the carotid artery of a client to determine whether chest compression is necessary. Which of the following actions should the nurse perform to assess the carotid artery?

   a. Use the heel of one hand

   b. Use two fingers

   c. Use the hands with locked elbows

   d. Use the jaw-thrust technique

10. A nurse needs to perform rescue breathing on a client with a laryngectomy. Which of the following actions should the nurse perform during rescue breathing?

    a. Seal the client's nose with the fingers

    b. Use a one-way valve mask

    c. Cover the client's mouth with a hand

    d. Seal the client's stoma with the mouth

11. A nurse needs to perform the Heimlich maneuver on an infant who has partial obstruction resulting from aspiration of vomitus. The nurse is holding the infant prone with the head downward. Which of the following should be the nurse's next action?

    a. Use two fingers to give back thrusts.

    b. Use the heel of the hand to give five back blows.

    c. Alternate the client between supine and prone positions.

    d. Use finger sweeps to remove the obstruction from the throat.

12. After opening the partial airway obstruction of a client, a nurse needs to assess the spontaneous breathing pattern of a client. How can the nurse assess spontaneous breathing in the client?

    a. Observe for the rising and falling of the chest

    b. Check the pulse rate at the wrist

    c. Observe the mouth and nose for movement

    d. Observe the change in skin color

13. A physician has ordered a nurse to discontinue resuscitation attached to a client with cardiac arrest. Which of the following factors contribute toward the discontinuing of resuscitation? Select all that apply.

    a. Data obtained from blood gas results and electrolyte studies

    b. The client's condition deteriorates despite resuscitation efforts

    c. Rescuers and emergency service nurses are exhausted

    d. The client's family is against the use of resuscitation

    e. The age of the client and the diagnosis given to the client

14. A nurse is performing chest compression on a middle-age client with cardiac arrest. Which of the following actions should the nurse perform to deliver a straight-down motion with each compression?

    a. Use two fingers to thrust the chest

    b. Avoid interlocking the fingers

    c. Rock back and forth over the client

    d. Position the body over the hands

15. A nurse is assisting a client with symptoms of cardiac arrest within the health care facility premises. Which of the following actions should the nurse perform to provide early emergency services to the client?

    a. Alert the lead physician of emergency service

    b. Notify the switchboard operator for assistance

    c. Assess the client and then dial 911

    d. Describe the client's age and physical appearance

End-of-Life Care

SECTION I: LEARNING OBJECTIVES

- Define terminal illness.
- Name the five stages of dying.
- Describe two methods by which nurses can promote acceptance of death in dying clients.
- Define respite care.
- Discuss the philosophy of hospice care.
- List at least five aspects of terminal care.
- Name at least five signs of multiple organ failure.
- Explain why a discussion of organ donation must take place as expeditiously as possible after a client's death.
- Name three components of postmortem care.
- Discuss the benefit of grieving.
- Describe one sign that a person is resolving his or her grief.

SECTION II: ASSESSING YOUR UNDERSTANDING

Activity A *Fill in the blanks.*

1. A(n) _____ illness means a condition from which recovery is beyond reasonable expectation.

2. The term _____ is the concept of caring for terminally ill clients.

3. _____ involves the maintenance of an adequate fluid volume.

4. _____ is determined on the basis that breathing and circulation have ceased.

5. _____ is one of the last reflexes to disappear as death approaches.

6. A(n) _____ is an examination of the organs and tissues of a human body after death.

7. A(n) _____ is a person legally designated to investigate deaths that may not be the result of natural causes.

8. The _____ is a person who prepares the body for burial or cremation.

9. A person who cannot accept someone's death is in a state of pathologic or _____ grief.

10. Some survivors have _____ experiences such as seeing, hearing, or feeling the continued presence of the deceased.

Activity B *Consider the following figure.*

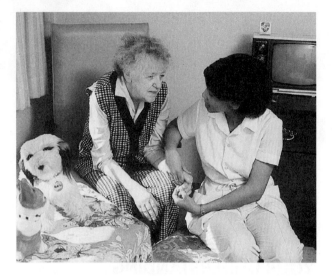

1. Identify the figure.

   _____

   _____

   _____

2. What are the responsibilities of the nurse in this kind of setup?

   _____

   _____

   _____

Activity C *Match the five stages of dying in column A with their descriptions in column B.*

Column A

____ **1.** Denial

____ **2.** Anger

____ **3.** Bargaining

____ **4.** Depression

____ **5.** Acceptance

Column B

A. Clients confront potential losses

B. Clients have dealt with their losses and have completed unfinished business

C. Clients retaliate against fate

D. Clients refuse to believe that the diagnosis is accurate

E. Clients are willing to accept death but want to extend their life temporarily

Activity D *Presented here, in random order, are the stages of grief. Write the correct sequence in the boxes provided.*

1. Developing awareness

2. Idealization

3. Shock and disbelief

4. Restitution period

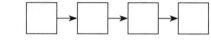

Activity E *Briefly answer the following.*

1. What does "dying with dignity" mean?

   _____

   _____

   _____

2. What is brain death?

   _____

   _____

   _____

3. What is a death certificate?

   _____

   _____

   _____

4. What is postmortem care?

   _____

   _____

   _____

5. What is multiple organ failure?

   _____

   _____

   _____

Activity F *Use the clues to complete the crossword puzzle.*

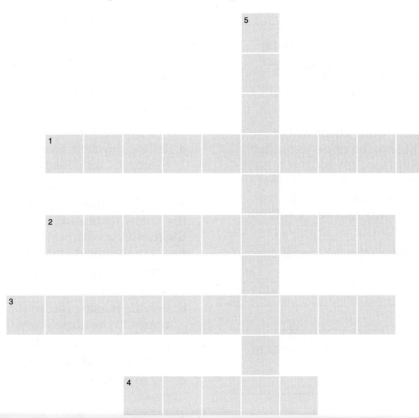

Across

1. These drugs have a pain-relieving property
2. Maintenance of an adequate fluid volume
3. Process of negotiation, usually with some higher power
4. Emotional response to feeling victimized

Down

5. Attitude of complacency

SECTION III: APPLYING YOUR KNOWLEDGE

Activity G *Nurses are more involved than any other group with people who experience impending death. Answer the following questions, which relate to a nurse's role in caring for a dying client.*

A nurse is caring for a young client with leukemia. The client asks the nurse to confirm if the laboratory reports are correct and to have them double-checked. The client is sure that there is a mistake, because all this happened while she was very healthy and active without any sign of illness.

1. What stage of dying is this client experiencing?

   _____

   _____

   _____

2. How should the nurse help dying clients to cope?

   _____

   _____

   _____

SECTION IV: PRACTICING FOR NCLEX

Activity H *Answer the following questions.*

1. A nurse is caring for a young client who has been severely injured in a motor vehicle accident. The client has multiple organ failure and is dying. Which of the following statements by the client indicates that the client is in the depression stage of dying?

   a. "How can it be? No, I'm not dying."

   b. "What have I done wrong? Why me?"

   c. "I have just finished college … ."

   d. "Yes, I'm dying … ."

2. A nurse is caring for an elderly client with a terminal illness. Which of the following interventions by the nurse indicates respect for the rights of the dying client?

   a. Asking the client to avoid talking about death

   b. Informing the client about preparing an advance directive

   c. Avoiding any reference to spirituality when talking to the client

   d. Telling the client that the results of the diagnostic test look good

3. A nurse is caring for an elderly client with acute renal failure who is dying. Which of the following nursing considerations must the nurse use when catering to the basic needs of the client and his family members?

   a. Offer to secure spiritual counseling, if requested, for the client and family members

   b. Provide nursing care to the client without regard to the nurse's own feelings

   c. Discourage the client from talking to family members about his death

   d. Try to convince the client and family members to agree to organ or tissue donation

4. A nurse is caring for a client with a terminal illness at her home. What interventions can the nurse offer to this client? Select all that apply.

   a. Coordinate community services

   b. Arrange for home nursing visits

   c. Secure home equipment

   d. Provide around-the-clock nursing care

   e. Suggest transferring the client to residential care

5. A nurse is caring for an elderly client with impaired swallowing. What care should the nurse take to prevent choking and aspiration in the client?

   a. Assist the client to a lateral position

   b. Ask the client to sleep without a pillow

   c. Assist the client to assume a semi-Fowler's position

   d. Ensure that the client is supine at all times

6. A client is admitted to the health care facility for a major surgery. The client has prepared an advance directive expressing his wish to donate his eyes in case of his death. The client died before the surgery. Which of the following should the nurse keep in mind when caring for the client's body?

   a. Harvest the eyes as soon as possible based on the client's directive

   b. Avoid placing hot or cold compresses over the client's eyes

   c. Avoid discussing the organ donation with the client's family members

   d. Discuss the possibility of harvesting the eyes after death with the client's next of kin

7. A nurse is caring for a terminally ill client who has been referred for hospice care. Which of the following clients are eligible for hospice care?

   a. Clients with less than 6 months to live

   b. Clients with difficult behavior

   c. Clients requiring high-tech palliative care

   d. Clients who cannot live independently

8. A client with carcinoma of the lung is receiving hospice care at her home. Which of the following are the services offered by hospice care?

   a. The client receives subacute or intermediate care

   b. The client is provided with labor-intensive treatment

   c. Around-the-clock nursing care is provided to the client

   d. Care is provided by a multidisciplinary team of professionals

9. A nurse is caring for an elderly client with impaired swallowing. What care should the nurse take to maintain adequate fluid volume in the client?

   a. Offer frequent small sips of water

   b. Offer small amounts of beverages

   c. Provide wrapped ice cubes to be sucked

   d. Inform the physician of the need for intravenous fluids

10. A nurse is caring for a client with bone cancer. The nurse identifies the risk of inadequate consumption of food. Which of the following are possible causes for this diagnosis?

    a. Pressure sores

    b. Nausea

    c. Weakness

    d. Infection

11. A nurse is caring for client who is terminally ill and prescribed oxygen therapy. Which of the following interventions is important for the client on oxygen therapy?

    a. Need for intravenous fluids

    b. Need for total parenteral nutrition

    c. Need for lubrication of the lips

    d. Need for frequent mouth care

12. A client with acute renal failure is administered non-narcotic analgesics. The nurse caring for this client is aware that which of the following is the goal of non-narcotic analgesics?

    a. To dull the consciousness

    b. To suppress respirations

    c. To inhibit the ability to communicate

    d. To provide relief from pain

13. A nurse is caring for an elderly client who has slipped into a coma. The client is showing signs of multiple organ failure. What care should the nurse take when summoning the family of the dying client? Select all that apply.

    a. Identify him- or herself by name, title, and location

    b. Ask the family to rush to the facility without explaining

    c. Ask for the family member by name and speak calmly

    d. Explain that the client's condition is deteriorating

    e. Tell the family all answers to queries will be given at the facility

14. A nurse is caring for a dying client who is in coma. Which of the following indicate brain death in the client? Select all that apply.

    a. Flat encephalogram for at least 10 minutes

    b. Unreceptiveness or unresponsiveness to moderately painful stimuli

    c. $PaCO_2$ less than 60 mm Hg after preoxygenation with 100% oxygen

    d. Complete absence of central and deep tendon reflexes

    e. No spontaneous respiration after being disconnected from a ventilator

15. A client at the health care facility has died after a prolonged illness. A nurse is assigned to perform postmortem care for the client. Which of the following interventions should the nurse perform when providing postmortem care?

    a. Clean secretions from the skin

    b. Remove dentures from the mouth

    c. Keep all hairpins and clips

    d. Place a rolled towel under the head

NOTES

NOTES

NOTES

NOTES